Diagnostic and Therapeutic Neuroradiology

João Xavier
Cristiana Vasconcelos
Cristina Ramos

Editors

Diagnostic and Therapeutic Neuroradiology

A Case-Based Guide to Good Practice

Foreword by Mario Muto

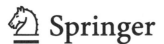 Springer

Introduction

What Is Neuroradiology?

As with most medical specialities, neuro-radiology has faintly defined borders. Of course there is a «core business»: to provide relevant images of the central nervous system in order to allow diagnostic and therapeutic procedures. However, other fields are usually added, «head and neck» being the generic designation for most of those areas. Between neuroradiology and radiology and between neuroradiology and neurology, neurosurgery or vascular surgery, there are some «no man's lands» which are either abandoned by everybody or which are fought over by many.

Instead, perhaps neuroradiology could best be defined by a principle that I heard many years ago from a first-generation neuroradiologist and founder of my department: «Neuroradiology is the deepest effort to reach the diagnosis of neurological diseases». Of course, this sentence must be considered in a broad sense. The key expression is «the deepest effort to reach», which may either be applied to diagnosis or therapeutics, not only to the strict field of neurological diseases, as mentioned above.

The purpose of this book is to show how real neuroradiology happens nowadays in high-activity neuroradiology departments. This is achieved by presenting illustrative clinical cases in diagnostic and therapeutic fields. The cases are presented in a quiz format: on the first page, the relevant clinical and image data are provided, leading to a few questions concerning image findings and differential diagnosis; on the back page, the solution is given and an explanation and short discussion are presented, as well as the relevant literature. This method allows the reader to learn about neuroradiology from studying real cases, reviewing the main pathologies and areas of interest in neuroradiology.

Parallel to the study of cases, the neuro-radiologist should also develop a solid clinical knowledge, at least at the level of neurological examination and neurological syndromes, as well as an updated technical knowledge about medical image media and familiarity with devices that can be used under image control, with more or less accuracy, according to the kind of procedures he or she is performing.

To present medical devices here is absolutely out of the question, as they are both too many and are constantly changing. To present the sequence of a neurological examination or to describe the neurological syndromes is also out of the scope of this introduction, in spite of the clinical data that are regularly provided in the cases we have selected. However, let us take a little walk through the medical imaging techniques and their applications in neuroradiology. Bear in mind that the different modalities of medical imaging must always distinguish between normal and pathological tissues by means of their different physical properties. Moreover, tomographic techniques (computed tomography, ultrasonography, magnetic resonance) take the properties of a «voxel» (volume element) to build up a «pixel» (picture element).

X-Ray Techniques

These techniques use a kind of ionising radiation (meaning radiation that can ionise atoms, thus damaging biological tissues), the X-rays, seeking their different attenuation in different materials. On computed tomography, the measure of that attenuation (the attenuation coefficient of each tissue) is usually converted to a more friendly number, the CT number or Hounsfield unit.

Plain X-ray images, computed tomography and angiography raise serious concerns about radiation dose. Unfortunately, nobody, besides a few conscientious doctors, pays much attention to this issue. So, neuroradiologists and other radiation professionals must be very cautious when using these kinds of techniques. Their potential harmful effect must always be balanced against the expected benefit they can provide. Although this is a common rule that should be applied to every medical image (as well as to other medical procedures, of course), it is especially crucial when using X-rays. The ALARA rule for radiation dose and number of images should always be kept in mind: as low as reasonably achievable.

Plain X-Ray Imaging

Do not underestimate plain X-ray images! They are cheap and fast and, at least for the spine, they are as yet the best widely available tool for studying static and dynamic balances. There is a wide range of lines and angles the neuroradiologist should learn elsewhere. Plain X-ray images can also provide prompt, accurate and almost direct information on osteo-articular degenerative and traumatic diseases. As they are poorly processed, X-ray images are very comprehensive images. One only needs to bear in mind the superimposition principle: do not forget that what you see on the image may lie anywhere along the X-ray beam path, including outside the body!

Angiography

Angiography allowed the first in vivo insight into the soft tissues inside the skull, and, in this sense, it is the root of neuroradiology. Younger doctors may not realise that angiography was used to diagnose brain tumours or haematomas, by correlating vessels shift with clinical data! But this was the aim which Dr. António Caetano Abreu Freire (don't you know this name?! Actually, this is the real name of Egas Moniz – do you recognise it now?) announced when he first presented this technique. Nowadays, CT scan and magnetic resonance imaging (MRI) can achieve this objective more easily whilst providing more information. However, angiography is still the gold standard for the sharp characterisation of vascular morphology and pathology and is also the main tool of interventional neuroradiology.

Usually, neuroangiography is performed under digital subtraction. This technique digitally removes the dense structures (the skull bones) already present before the introduction of contrast medium, allowing better visualisation of the soft tissues that contain contrast medium, mainly vessels. Being an «enhanced» X-ray image, angiography is also a comprehensive image, made even clearer when a biplanar suite is available, with which one can see two projections in real time. Moreover, modern angiography suites combine the conventional digital subtraction angiography technique with CT techniques, allowing 3D reformatting, multiplanar imaging and volume rendering. These tools are especially useful when complex vascular lesions or extravascular interventional complications are to be seen.

Angiography demands practical skills as well as theoretical knowledge. The neuroradiologist has to learn how to move catheters and guidewires in order to reach the vessel he or she is trying to see by means of a local injection of iodine contrast medium, to promptly recognise alterations and to customise the procedure as these alterations are detected. Of course, the interventional neuroradiologist also has to choose the appropriate therapeutics and know how to use the several available devices.

Computed Tomography (CT Scan)

Although MRI is becoming more widespread, CT is still the first tool of the neuroradiologist, especially in the emergency room.

V   Vascular

VI   Degenerative Diseases

VII   Spine

VIII   Metabolic and Toxic Diseases

Contribu[

Luís Albuquerq
Neuroradiology D
Centro Hospitalar
Porto, Portugal
luis.pinheiro87@g

Ricardo Almen
Neurology Depart
Centro Hospitalar
Trás-os-Montes e
Alto Douro, Portug
ricardo.jorge.alme

José Eduardo A
Neuroradiology D
Centro Hospitalar
Porto, Portugal
zeedualves@gmail

Viriato Alves
Neuroradiology D
Centro Hospitalar
Porto, Portugal
viriatoalves@mac.

Gonçalo Basílio
Neuroimaging Dep
Northern Lisbon H
Lisbon, Portugal
goncalobasilio@hc

Fidel Bastos
Department of Rac
Sagrada Esperança
Luanda, Angola
bastoscastro@hotr

Teresa Bernardo
Department of Inte
Sagrada Esperança
Luanda, Angola
teresa.bernardo86@

Luís Botelho
Neuroradiology, Ne
Neurosurgery Depa
Centro Hospitalar d
Porto, Portugal

Alexandre Mendes
Neuroradiology, Neurology and
Neurosurgery Departments
Centro Hospitalar do Porto
Porto, Portugal
falexandremendes@gmail.com

Bruno Moreira
Neuroradiology Department
Centro Hospitalar do Porto
Porto, Portugal
brunoic2@gmail.com

Mario Muto
Neuroradiology Service
Cardarelli Hospital
Naples, Italy
mutomar@tiscali.it

Lia Neto
Neuroimaging Department
Northern Lisbon Hospital Centre
Lisbon, Portugal
lia_neto@yahoo.com

Joana Nunes
Department of Imaging, Neuroradiology
Centro Hospitalar Vila Nova de Gaia/Espinho
Espinho, Portugal
joanita_bgc@hotmail.com

Cláudia Pereira
Neuroradiology Department
Centro Hospitalar do Porto
Porto, Portugal
claudiamsspereira@gmail.com

Daniela Jardim Pereira
Centro Hospitalar e Universitário de Coimbra
Coimbra, Portugal
danielajardimpereira@gmail.com

José Pedro Rocha Pereira
Neuroradiology Department
Centro Hospitalar do Porto
Porto, Portugal
jprochapereira@gmail.com

Sofia Pina
Neuroradiology Department
Centro Hospitalar do Porto
Porto, Portugal
docsofia@gmail.com

Carolina Pinheiro
Neuroradiology Department
Centro Hospitalar de Lisboa Central
Lisbon, Portugal
carolinafpinheiro@gmail.com

Joana T. Pinto
Neuroradiology Department
Centro Hospitalar e Universitário de Coimbra
Coimbra, Portugal
joanatpinto@hotmail.com

Pedro Pinto
Neuroradiology Department
Centro Hospitalar do Porto
Porto, Portugal
p@pinto.as

Vasco Pinto
Department of Neurosurgery
Centro Hospitalar do Porto
Porto, Portugal
vascosapinto@gmail.com

Manuel Melo Pires
Centro Hospitalar do Porto
Unit of Neuropathology
Porto, Portugal
melopires@hotmail.com

Daniela Prayer
Neuroradiology Department
Medical University of Vienna
Vienna, Austria
daniela.prayer@meduniwien.ac.at

Cristina Ramos
Neuroradiology Department
Centro Hospitalar do Porto
Porto, Portugal
crisgiesta@gmail.com

Inês Rego
Imagiology Department
Centro Hospitalar de Trás-os-
Montes e Alto Douro
Alto Douro, Portugal
i.cabralrego@gmail.com

Sofia Reimão
Department of Neuroimaging
Hospital de Santa Maria
Lisbon, Portugal
sofiapcr@gmail.com

Valentina Ribeiro
Neuroradiology Department
Centro Hospitalar do Porto
Porto, Portugal
valentina.ribeiro97@gmail.com

André Rodrigues
Internal Medicine Department
Northern Lisbon Hospital Centre
Lisbon, Portugal
rodrigues87andre@gmail.com

Marta Rodrigues
Department of Imaging, Neuroradiology
Centro Hospitalar Vila Nova de Gaia/Espinho
Espinho , Portugal
marta56169@gmail.com

Tiago Rodrigues
Neuroradiology Departments
Centro Hospitalar do Funchal and Centro
Hospitalar do Porto
Funchal and Porto, Portugal
tyagorodrigues@gmail.com

Maria Goreti Sá
Neuroradiology Department
Centro Hospitalar do Porto
Porto, Portugal
mariagoretisa@gmail.com

Carla Silva
Neuroradiology, Neurology and
Neurosurgery Departments
Centro Hospitalar do Porto
Porto, Portugal
carlaestevessilva@hotmail.com

Nuno Ferreira Silva
Neuroradiology Department
Centro Hospitalar do Porto
Porto, Portugal
fsnuno@sapo.pt

Ricardo Taipa
Centro Hospitalar do Porto
Porto, Portugal
ricardotaipa@gmail.com

Joana Tavares
Department of Neuroimaging
Hospital de Santa Maria
Lisbon, Portugal

Neuroimaging Department
Northern Lisbon Hospital Centre
Porto, Portugal
joanabaratatavares@gmail.com

João Teixeira
Neuroradiology Department
Centro Hospitalar do Porto
Porto, Portugal
joaofcteixeira@gmail.com

Cristiana Vasconcelos
Neuroradiology Department
Centro Hospitalar do Porto
Porto, Portugal
cjpvasconcelos@yahoo.com

Marcos Gil da Veiga
Neuroradiology Department
Centro Hospitalar de Lisboa Central
Lisbon, Portugal
neuroradiology.veiga@gmail.com

António Verdelho
Neurosurgery Department
Instituto Português de Oncologia do Porto
Porto, Portugal
verdelho.netc@gmail.com

Pedro Viana
Neurology Department
Hospital de Santa Maria – Centro
Hospitalar Lisboa Norte
Lisbon, Portugal
pedrofaroviana@gmail.com

Nuno Vila-Chã
Neuroradiology, Neurology and
Neurosurgery Departments
Centro Hospitalar do Porto
Porto, Portugal
nunovilacha@hotmail.com

João Xavier
Neuroradiology Department
Centro Hospitalar do Porto
Porto, Portugal
director.neurorradiologia@hgsa.min-saude.pt

Case 1

Adalgisa Dias, Valentina Ribeiro, and Cristina Ramos

© Springer International Publishing AG 2018
J. Xavier et al. (eds.), *Diagnostic and Therapeutic Neuroradiology*,
https://doi.org/10.1007/978-3-319-61140-2_1

1

A 16-week-old child with a history of intrauterine growth restriction, currently with delayed cognitive growth and epilepsy (◘ Figs. 1.1, 1.2, 1.3 and 1.4)

❓ Questions

1. What are the findings on these MR images?
2. What are the differential diagnoses?
3. How is the diagnosis made?

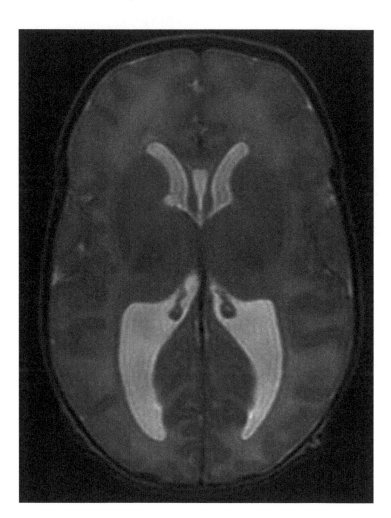

◘ **Fig. 1.1** Axial T2

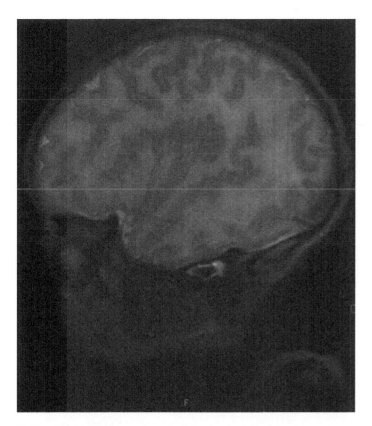

◘ Fig. 1.2   Sagittal T2

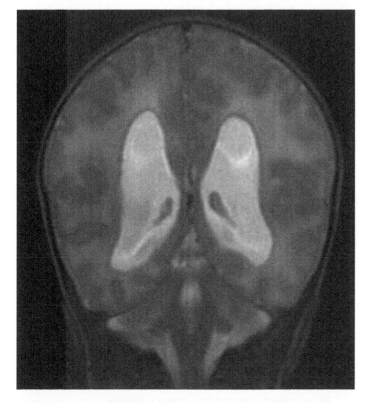

◘ Fig. 1.3   Coronal T2

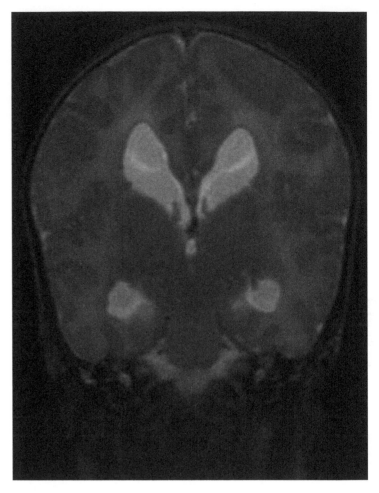

Fig. 1.4 Coronal T2

Diagnosis   Bilateral perisylvian polymicrogyria

✅ **Answers to Questions**
1. On MRI, there are periventricular germinolytic cysts, more prominent on the right, moderate enlargement of the lateral ventricles (ventriculomegaly) of 14 mm and bilateral perisylvian polymicrogyria.
2. Differential diagnoses include lissencephaly, pachygyria and other cortical malformations.
3. The diagnosis is typically made by magnetic resonance imaging (MRI) that reveals either irregularity of the cortical surface, suggestive of multiple small folds, or an irregular, scalloped appearance of the grey matter-white matter junction. The cerebral cortex often appears abnormally thick. Polymicrogyria can result from both genetic and environmental causes and can occur as an isolated finding with no other systemic involvement or as part of a syndrome with multisystem involvement. To date, the only gene known to be associated with polymicrogyria is GPR56.

1.1   Comments

Polymicrogyria is a malformation of cortical development that is characterised by abnormal arrangement and excessive folding of cerebral cortical cell layers, often with fusion of the gyral surfaces. It is thought to result from abnormal organisation of neurons within the cortical lamina after completion of neuroblast migration from the germinal zone and through the intermediate zone of the developing brain [1].

Polymicrogyria can result from intrauterine infection (e.g. cytomegalovirus, toxoplasmosis, syphilis and varicella zoster virus); and intrauterine ischemia (as in twin-twin transfusion) [2].

It can occur as an isolated finding with no other systemic involvement or as part of a syndrome with multisystem involvement.

The diagnosis of polymicrogyria is typically made by magnetic resonance imaging (MRI) since computed tomography (CT) and other imaging methods generally do not have high enough resolution or adequate contrast to identify the small folds that define the condition. In particular, MRI can demonstrate an irregularity of the cortical surface suggestive of multiple small folds or an irregular, scalloped appearance to the grey matter-white matter junction, the latter often being more evident.

Polymicrogyria is usually isolated but can also be seen in association with other brain malformations. In certain malformations, such as schizencephaly, polymicrogyria is almost invariably present (in this case, along the cleft that connects the ventricle to the brain surface). The association of polymicrogyria with grey matter heterotopia, agenesis of the corpus callosum, and other developmental brain anomalies has been reported [1, 2].

References

1. James Barkovich A, Hevner R, Guerrini R. Syndromes of bilateral symmetrical Polymicrogyria. AJNR Am J Neuroradiol. 1999;20:1814–21.
2. A. James Barkovich. Current concepts of polymicrogyria. Neuroradiology. University of California at San Francisco. 2010; 52:479–87.

Case 2

Otília Marrime Farrão and José Eduardo Alves

© Springer International Publishing AG 2018
J. Xavier et al. (eds.), *Diagnostic and Therapeutic Neuroradiology*,
https://doi.org/10.1007/978-3-319-61140-2_2

A 1-day-old baby is born through emergent C-section at 36 weeks of gestational age due to sudden signs of fetal distress. At birth, he presented bleeding from the umbilical stump and epistaxis. Apgar score was 3/6, with the need for mechanical ventilation. There is familiar history of one brother deceased after birth due to prenatal brain bleeding of uncertain etiology and another healthy brother. Initial platelet count and coagulation screening tests were normal.

❓ Questions

1. Describe the imaging findings in A and B.
2. What does the lesion in C (white arrow) suggest?
3. Taking into account the clinical information and ultrasound, what would be your main differential diagnosis?

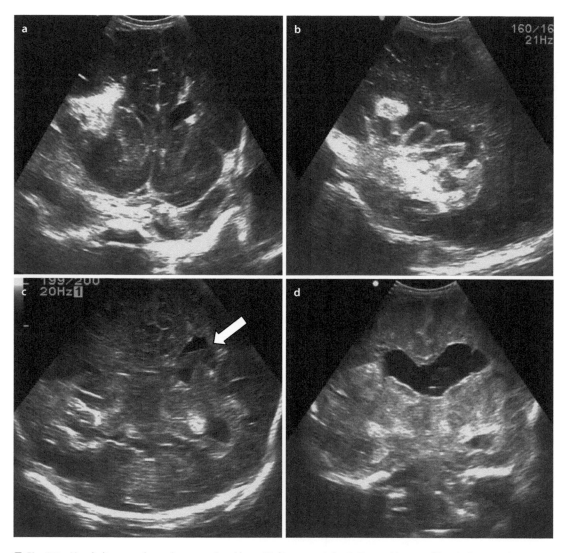

⬚ Fig. 2.1 Head ultrasound **a** and **c** coronal and **b** sagittal images at day 1. Coronal image of head ultrasound performed at day 7 **d**

Diagnosis   Congenital factor XIII deficiency

✓ **Answers**

1. Bilateral acute/recent parenchymal hemorrhagic lesions, without evidence of intraventricular blood. The one on the right has ruptured to the subarachnoid space.
2. Left hemisphere old periventricular lesion, with cavitation and marked irregularity of the ventricular contour.
3. Congenital bleeding disorders, including vasculopathies, coagulopathies, and metabolic disorders.

2.1   Comments

Congenital FXIII deficiency is a rare genetic bleeding disorder, with an estimated prevalence of 1 case per 2–3 million individuals. It affects males and females equally and is inherited as an autosomal recessive trait.

The symptoms of factor XIII deficiency have variable severity and may become apparent at any age, although most cases are identified during infancy. Common symptoms include bleeding from the umbilical stump, epistaxis, muscle hematoma, subcutaneous bleeding, and high risk of miscarriage. About one third of patients present intracerebral bleeding, a risk greater than in other related bleeding disorders and the leading cause of mortality [1].

The diagnosis of this disorder is a challenge, not only due to its rarity but also because typical coagulation screening and platelet function tests are normal.

Intracranial hemorrhage in neonates is not a rare finding and can occur as a result of prematurity, birth trauma, platelet disorders (congenital, alloimmune), coagulation disorders, infections, and hypoxia.

In this case, the relevant familiar history and the presence of brain lesions of different ages (◼ Fig. 2.1a and c) suggested a genetic inherited etiology. Differential diagnoses include congenital coagulopathies and vasculopathies but also some metabolic diseases, such as congenital disorders of glycosylation and mitochondrial respiratory chain defects.

Reference

1. Bertamino M, et al. Diagnosis and management of severe congenital factor XIII deficiency in the emergent department. Blood Transfus. 2015;13:324–7.

Case 3

Valentina Ribeiro

© Springer International Publishing AG 2018
J. Xavier et al. (eds.), *Diagnostic and Therapeutic Neuroradiology*,
https://doi.org/10.1007/978-3-319-61140-2_3

Screening sonography of the 28-week-old fetus of a woman revealed a homogeneous and solid anterior neck mass.

? **Questions**

1. Where is the lesion?
2. What is the differential diagnosis?
3. What could be the cause?

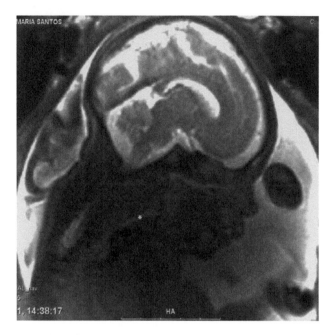

◘ **Fig. 3.1**   Sagital T2; *pointing trachea

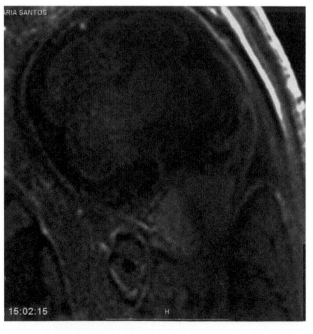

◘ **Fig. 3.2**   Coronal T1

Diagnostic Fetal goiter

✅ **Answers**

1. Sagittal T2 (◘ Fig. 3.1) shows hypointense mass surrounding fluid-filled trachea (*). Coronal T1 shows hyperintense bilobate mass consistent with goiter (◘ Fig. 3.2).
2. Teratoma, lymphangioma, hemangioma, neuroblastoma, and rhabdomyoma.
3. Autoimmune thyroid disease is common in pregnancy. Graves' disease is present in about 0.2% of pregnancies. Antibodies to the thyroid-stimulating hormone receptor (TSH-R) freely cross the placenta and can act in the fetal thyroid gland during the second half of pregnancy.

3.1 Comments

Fetal goiter is an enlargement of the thyroid gland in utero. It can occur with hyper- or hypothyroidism.

It occurs in 8% of fetuses of hyperthyroid mothers in antithyroid therapy and manifests as a symmetric homogeneous solid bilobed anterior neck mass on sonography after the fetal thyroid begins to function late in the first trimester [1].

Fetal goiter may result in significant complications at delivery due to airway obstruction, including hypoxic-ischemic brain injury and death [1].

Polyhydramnios due to poor fetal swallowing indicates potential airway obstruction and should prompt MR imaging.

Thyroid T2 signal intensity varies with functional status, hypointense if protein, and iodine concentration is high and hyperintense if they are low. T1 hyperintensity is more consistent [1], and an associated bilobate shape is pathognomonic of fetal goiter [2].

References

1. Letters. AJNR 32. 2011.
2. Hernandez MI, Lee KK-W. Neonatal Graves disease caused by transplacental antibodies. NeoReviews. 2008;9:e305.

Case 4

Delfina Covini, Mariana C. Diogo, and Daniela Prayer

© Springer International Publishing AG 2018
J. Xavier et al. (eds.), *Diagnostic and Therapeutic Neuroradiology*,
https://doi.org/10.1007/978-3-319-61140-2_4

A 22-year old pregnant woman without known pathologies was referred for fetal MRI due to abnormal findings on the 31 gestational weeks (GW) prenatal ultrasound. Brain, heart, and digestive tract anomalies were suspected. Fetal MRI was performed at 31 + 2 GW and postmortem at 32 GW.

? Questions
1. What are the findings on these MR images?
2. What is the most likely etiology?
3. What should be imaged next?

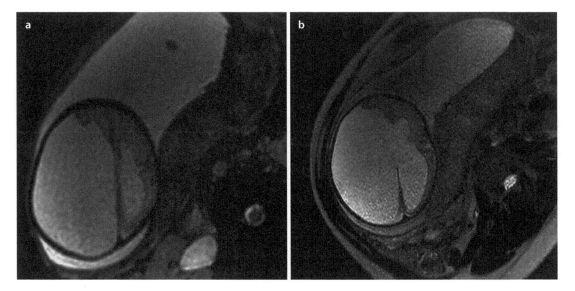

◻ Fig. 4.1   Fetal MRI at 32 GW **a** axial T2EPI and **b** axial T2SSFSE

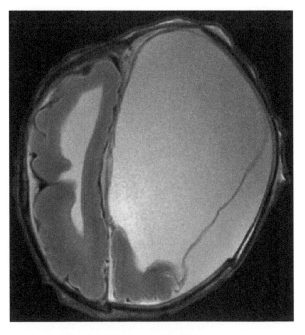

◻ Fig. 4.2   Postmortem MRI high-resolution T2WI

Diagnosis   Hydrocephalus and schizencephaly due to fetal vascular disruption

✅ **Answers to Questions**

1. Axial T2WI shows massive hydrocephalus, with asymmetrical supratentorial ventricular dilatation and any residual brain parenchyma in the right parietal, temporal, and occipital lobe regions. There are schizencephaly clefts bilaterally (◘ Figs. 4.1a, b and 4.2).
2. Most likely etiology is vascular disruption. Notice there is a schizencephaly cleft in the right hemisphere as well (◘ Figs. 4.1a, b and 4.2).
3. Placental imaging. The posterior placenta shows a non-age-related signal behavior with T2 inhomogeneous signal (◘ Fig. 4.1a, b).

4.1   Comments

This case demonstrates not only the potential of prenatal MRI to detect fetal brain anomalies but also that it is possible to overlook some brain injuries when this imaging method is used at advanced gestational ages. In cases such as this, not only the brain but also the placenta should be looked at, considering that we are faced with the final imaging result of a probable vascular disruption process. It is known that prenatal vascular events may disrupt fetal structures, creating a variety of congenital anomalies [1]. In early vascular disruption events, brain lesions such as schizencephaly may occur. After this initial event, bleeding originates aqueduct obstruction, finally resulting in severe supratentorial hydrocephaly. It is important to consider that many of the brain lesions could be due to vascular injuries and consequent disruptive process and not only be the consequence of genetic alterations or abnormal embryogenesis [2].

References

1. Howe DT, Rankin J, Draper ES. Schizencephaly prevalence, prenatal diagnosis and clues to etiology: a register-based study. Ultrasound Obstet Gynecol. 2012;39:75–82.
2. Lubinsky MS. Hypothesis: septo-optic dysplasia is a vascular disruption sequence. Am J Med Genet. 1997;69:235–6.

Case 5

José Eduardo Alves

© Springer International Publishing AG 2018
J. Xavier et al. (eds.), *Diagnostic and Therapeutic Neuroradiology*,
https://doi.org/10.1007/978-3-319-61140-2_5

Two-day-old girl, second-born twin of a dichorionic diamniotic pregnancy. Born 1h later than the first twin through emergent C-section at 39 weeks of gestational age due to breech presentation, Apgar score 1/4/6 (1, 5, 10 min). Presented severe hypotonia and clonic movements of the right hand. Ultrasound performed at day 2 and MR at day 10.

❓ Questions

1. What are the imaging findings in A and B?
2. What is the diagnosis?
3. If no intervention is planned, what is the optimal time for early MR imaging?

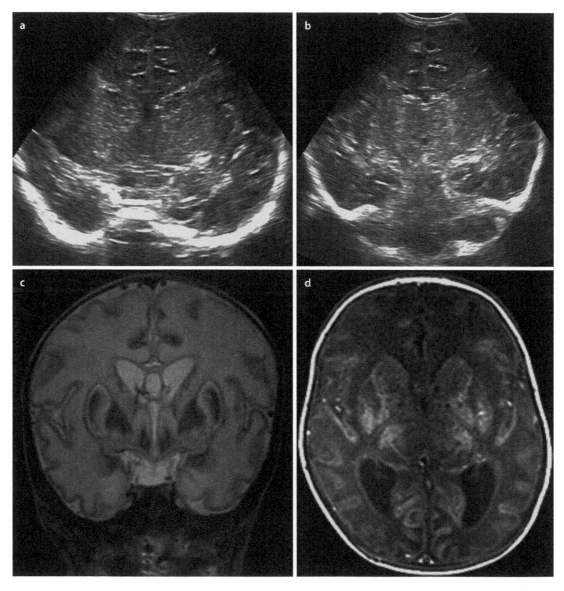

◻ **Fig. 5.1** Head ultrasound **a** and **b** coronal images performed at age 3 days. MRI **c** coronal T2 TSE and **d** axial T1 images at age 10 days

Diagnosis   Severe hypoxic-ischemic injury

✅ **Answers**
1. Diffuse hyperechogenicity of the deep grey nuclei and white matter
2. Perinatal hypoxic-ischemic injury
3. Three to five days postnatal

5.1   Comments

Most hypoxic-ischemic (HI) brain injury in neonates results from cerebral hypoperfusion. The pattern of neonatal brain injury and the final prognosis depends mainly on the severity and duration of the hypoperfusion event and the maturity of the brain at the time of injury.

Thus, term neonates with severe HI encephalopathy will suffer damage firstly to the most metabolically active and mature regions of the brain, namely, the lateral thalami, posterior putamina, subthalamic nuclei, hippocampi and corticospinal tracts. In extremely severe cases, such as this one, there may also be diffuse involvement of the cortex, white matter and brainstem, the prognosis being very poor.

Imaging findings evolve continuously during the first weeks, so the timing at which studies are performed is crucial for a correct assessment.

In the first few days, ultrasound shows progressive hyperechogenicity, mainly in the deep grey nuclei, periventricular white matter and perirolandic cortex (◧ Fig. 5.1a and b). Transcranial Doppler might show decreased resistive index due to impaired autoregulation.

Diffusion-weighted imaging is the most sensitive MR sequence in the first 48–72 h but will likely underestimate the amount of damage if performed in the first 24 h. Between 3 and 5 days after injury, T1-, and T2-weighted images will start depicting hyperintense lesions and diffusion abnormalities will be at their maximum. Proton MRS will show elevated lactate and diminished NAA peaks [1].

Reference

1. Barkovich AJ. Pediatric Neuroimaging. 5th ed. Philadelphia: Wolters Kluwer Health/Lippincott Williams & Wilkins; 2012.

Case 6

João Teixeira

© Springer International Publishing AG 2018
J. Xavier et al. (eds.), *Diagnostic and Therapeutic Neuroradiology*,
https://doi.org/10.1007/978-3-319-61140-2_6

36-year-old female with left facial naevus, right hemiparesis and epilepsy

❓ Questions
1. What is the clinical diagnosis?
2. What is missing and what is unexpected with regard to the imaging?
3. Which other diagnosis can be proposed by the imaging?

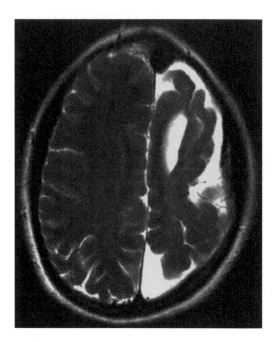

◘ Fig. 6.1   Axial T2

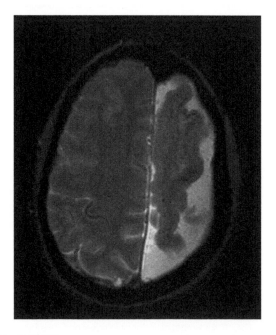

◘ Fig. 6.2   Axial T2*

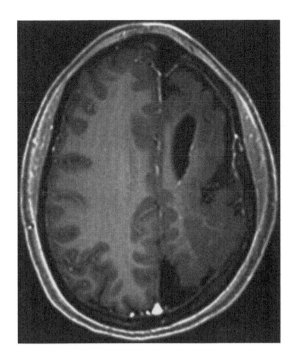

Fig. 6.3   Axial T1 with gadolinium

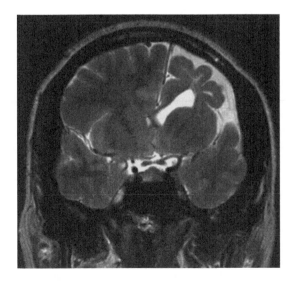

Fig. 6.4   Coronal T2

Diagnosis   Sturge-Weber syndrome with polymicrogyria

✔ **Answers to Questions**
1. Sturge-Weber syndrome (SWS).
2. T2-WI and T2*-WI imaging (◘ Figs. 6.1 and 6.2) show atrophy and subcortical calcification in the left cerebral hemisphere, expected in SWS. However, the typical leptomeningeal enhancement, the most characteristic finding, is missing (◘ Fig. 6.3).
3. MRI depicts cortical anomaly in frontal and Sylvian regions that can be classified as polymicrogyria. Coronal T2-WI (◘ Fig. 6.4) shows the cortical malformation in another plan, with abnormally thick cortex, although it could be misinterpreted as atrophy.

6.1   Comments

Sturge-Weber syndrome (SWS), also known as encephalotrigeminal angiomatosis, is a rare, sporadic, congenital, neurocutaneous syndrome characterized by facial naevus, ipsilateral leptomeningeal angiomatosis, and ophthalmologic abnormalities (such as congenital glaucoma and haemangiomas of the choroid) [1].

The most common neurological features are epileptic seizures, cognitive impairment, and hemiparesis.

Although the diagnosis of SWS is often straightforward on the basis of dermatological and neurological findings, demonstration of the pial abnormality on contrast-enhanced MRI (the most important criterion for the imaging diagnosis) could be helpful.

However, in some cases there is a regression of the leptomeningeal enhancement over time, as the cortex has been reduced to a nonfunctioning calcified mantle and is no longer perfused, as seen in this case [2].

Previously thought of as rare, cortical malformations are consistently identified in patients with SWS, evaluated for epilepsy surgery. Clinical presentation in this subgroup could be severe, with medically intractable seizures, and associated with cognitive and motor deficits [1].

The association of SWS with cortical malformations, including polymicrogyria and focal cortical dysplasia, is not so rare in patients with medically intractable epilepsy and Sturge-Weber syndrome, and a cortical malformation could be a significant contributor to severe neurological presentation [3].

Early ischemic in utero insults may be the genesis of cortical malformations, thought to be acquired during the second trimester.

The finding of SWS can mask the cortical malformation under atrophy and increased signal intensities on T2WI.

Complete resection of these cortical malformations, and not only resection of the angioma and underlying cortex, carry a better outcome of epilepsy surgery. On the contrary, if the cortical malformation remains unrecognised under angiomatosis, the prognosis is worse as malformed cortex is more likely to constitute the epileptogenic zone.

Note: the patient was not submitted to surgery, and we do not have histological confirmation.

References

1. Maton B, Krsek P, Jayakar P, Resnick T, Koehn M, Morrison G, et al. Medically intractable epilepsy in Sturge-Weber syndrome is associated with cortical malformation: implications for surgical therapy. Epilepsia. 2010;51(2): 257–67.
2. Fischbein NJ, Barkovich AJ, Wu Y, Berg BO. Sturge-Weber syndrome with no leptomeningeal enhancement on MRI. Neuroradiology. 1998;40(3):177–80.
3. Wang DD, Blümcke I, Coras R, Zhou WJ, Lu DH, Gui QP, et al. Sturge-Weber syndrome is associated with cortical dysplasia ILAE type IIIc and excessive hypertrophic pyramidal neurons in brain resections for intractable epilepsy. Brain Pathol. 2015;25(3):248–55.

Case 7

Cristiana Vasconcelos

© Springer International Publishing AG 2018
J. Xavier et al. (eds.), *Diagnostic and Therapeutic Neuroradiology*,
https://doi.org/10.1007/978-3-319-61140-2_7

A six-month-old female with craniofacial dysmorphia, third and fourth toe syndactyly and mutation in the TWIST1 gene.

? Questions
1. What are the findings?
2. Name the major suture synostosis types.
3. Classify this syndrome.

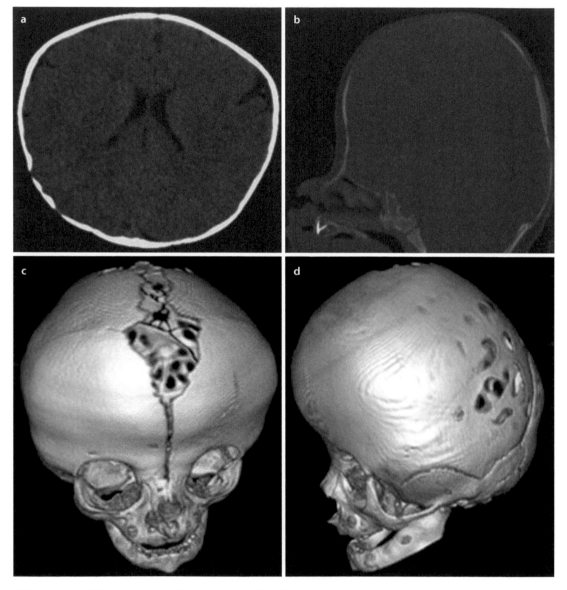

◘ **Fig. 7.1**   Axial HRCT images **a** with coronal **b** and 3D surface **c, d** reconstructions

Diagnosis   Saethre-Chotzen syndrome

✅ **Answers to Questions**

1. Bicoronal fusion (◻ Fig. 7.1a, b) resulting in brachycephaly with secondary upper and midface hypoplasia (◻ Fig. 7.1c, d).

2. Dolichocephaly/scaphocephaly (premature fusion of sagittal suture), brachycephaly (bicoronal fusion), anterior or posterior plagiocephaly (unicoronal or unilateral lambdoid fusion), trigonocephaly (metopic fusion), oxycephaly (combination of severe sagittal and coronal fusion) and Kleeblattschadel/cloverleaf (combined sagittal, coronal and lambdoid fusion).

3. Craniosynostosis and digital anomalies (syndactyly) characterise the acrocephalosyndactyly syndromes (ACS). The mutation in the TWIST 1 gene is associated with Saethre-Chotzen syndrome.

7.1   Comments

Primary craniosynostosis (premature fusion of cranial sutures) may be isolated (80–90%) or part of a larger syndrome. ACS comprise a rare group of disorders collectively characterised by craniosynostosis and fusion or webbing of the fingers or toes, often with other associated manifestations (skeletal defects, cardiac defect and other organ anomalies). Crouzon's, Apert's and Pfeiffer's syndromes are the most common craniofacial syndromes. The pattern of inheritance is autosomal dominant, but de novo mutations are very common. Mutations have been found in fibroblast growth factor receptor-1 (FGFR1), FGFR2 and FGFR3 (associated with Crouzon's, Apert's, Pfeiffer's, Beare-Stevenson, Jackson-Weiss and Muenke syndromes), twist homolog 1 (TWIST1) (associated with Saethre-Chotzen syndrome) and msh homeobox 2 (MSX2) genes (Boston-type craniosynostosis) [1].

Saethre-Chotzen syndrome affects males and females equally and has variable expressivity. These patients may have short stature, facial asymmetry, hypertelorism, ptosis, buphthalmos, beaked nose, deafness, radioulnar synostosis and cardiac defect.

Most individuals have normal intelligence, but mild to moderate intellectual disability is sometimes present.

When there is raised intracranial pressure and restriction of brain growth, surgical treatment is indicated and is most effective in the first year of life.

Deformational or positional plagiocephaly results from in utero flattening modulated, in the postnatal period, by preferential head position with infants sleeping on their backs. No synostosis is present in these cases.

Reference

1. Khanna PC, Thapa MM, Iyer RS, Prasad SS. Pictorial essay: the many faces of craniosynostosis. Indian J Radiol Imaging. 2011;21(1):49–56.

Case 8

João Jacinto, Catarina Perry da Câmara, and Carla Conceição

© Springer International Publishing AG 2018
J. Xavier et al. (eds.), *Diagnostic and Therapeutic Neuroradiology*,
https://doi.org/10.1007/978-3-319-61140-2_8

A 3-day-old newborn female was admitted to the hospital with stiffness of the left leg associated with heat and erythematous and vesicular rash. At 6 days old, seizures begin and the rash spreads through the body, being more intense on the face, limbs, and perianal region. There was no fever, mental status changes or other clinical signs. Previous personal history was uneventful, including the delivery. However, the mother had active lip herpes since before birth. Blood and CSF analysis were normal but transfontanelar ultrasound revealed periventricular and thalamic hyperechogenicity (◙ Figs. 8.1, 8.2, 8.3, and 8.4).

❓ Questions

1. What are the MRI findings?
2. What is the most probable diagnosis based only on clinical history and examination?
3. Excluding infectious diseases, which other pathology, or pathologies, should be included?

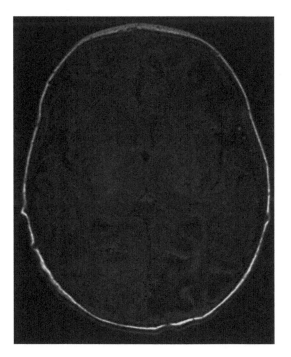

◙ **Fig. 8.1**   Axial T1

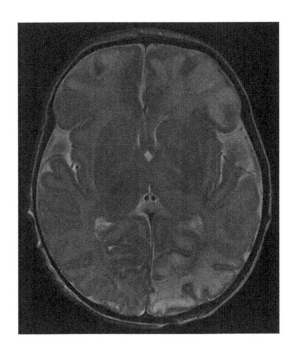

■ Fig. 8.2 Axial T2

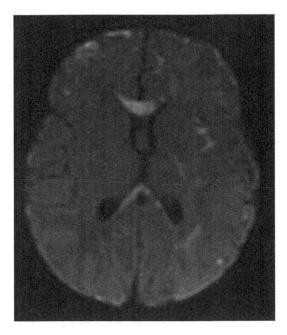

■ Fig. 8.3 DWI

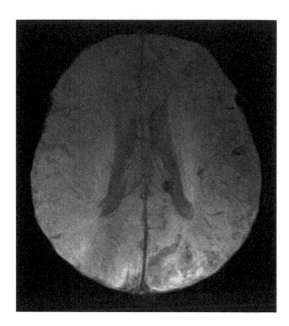

◘ **Fig. 8.4** SWI

Diagnosis   Incontinentia pigmenti (IP)

✅ **Answers to Questions**
1. Extensive multifocal cortical and subcortical acute lesions, involving both brain hemispheres, left thalamus, and corpus callosum, with laminar cortical necrosis and tumescent white matter changes, suggesting evolution to necrotic cavitation lesions.
2. Viral encephalitis.
3. Incontinentia pigmenti. Although commonly seen in viral encephalitis or sepsis, these cutaneous and MRI findings should include IP in the differential diagnosis.

8.1   Comments

IP is a rare neurocutaneous disorder which affects the CNS in 30–50% of cases [2]. The diagnosis is made by pathognomonic skin lesions appearing in four stages: erythematous and vesicular rash occurring at birth or early after, hyperkeratotic linear plaques, hyperpigmentation following Blaschko's lines, and dermal scarring. Neonatal IP presents only with the first stage lesions, which may also be seen in acute infectious diseases, making prompt diagnosis difficult. Acute CNS manifestations include abnormal signal mainly in the white matter, acute destructive lesions with edema, hemorrhagic foci, and necrotic cavitations, which evolve to parenchymal atrophy, including corpus callosum. Mental retardation, seizures, spastic paralysis, microcephaly, and cerebellar ataxia are common clinical symptoms. Treatment is symptomatic [1, 2].

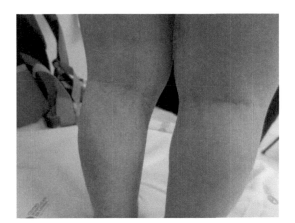

References

1. Castroviejo I, Ruggieri M. Chapter 18: Incontinentia Pigmenti. In: Neurocutaneous disorders. Germany: Springer; 2008. p. 391–404.
2. Wolf N, et al. Diffuse cortical necrosis in a neonate with incontinentia pigmenti and an encephalitis-like presentation. AJNR Am J Neuroradiol. 2005;26:1580–2.

Case 9

Marcos Gil da Veiga, Mariana Cardoso Diogo, and Carla Conceição

© Springer International Publishing AG 2018
J. Xavier et al. (eds.), *Diagnostic and Therapeutic Neuroradiology*,
https://doi.org/10.1007/978-3-319-61140-2_9

A 5-year-old girl was evacuated from Cape Verde for corrective surgery due to progressive scoliosis, noted by age 3. She was born at term to nonconsanguineous parents, after an uneventful pregnancy. At admission a complete absence of the horizontal eye movements was identified, with preserved convergence and vertical eye movements.

? Questions

1. What are the findings?
2. What is the differential diagnosis?
3. What other sequences/MR techniques would be useful?

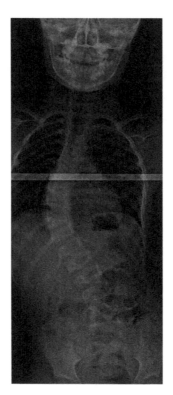

◨ Fig. 9.1   PA radiograph

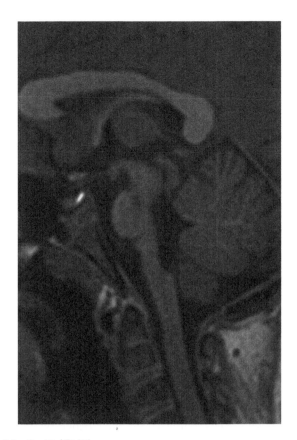

■ Fig. 9.2   Sagittal T1-WI

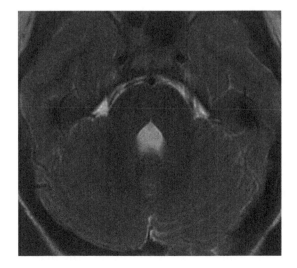

■ Fig. 9.3   Axial T2-WI

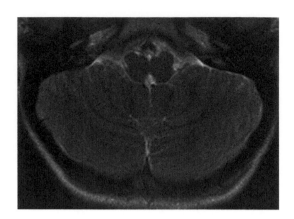

◘ Fig. 9.4   Axial T2-WI

Diagnosis   Horizontal gaze palsy with progressive scoliosis (HGPPS), ROBO3 positive

✅ **Answers to Questions**
1. Thoracolumbar scoliosis (◘ Fig. 9.1), pons and medulla hypoplasia (◘ Fig. 9.2) with butterfly-shaped medulla (◘ Fig. 9.4) and tent-shaped fourth ventricle (◘ Fig. 9.3), with absent facial colliculi
2. Differential diagnosis: Neurofibromatosis type 1, genetic disorders of eye control (Duane and Moebius syndromes)
3. Diffusion tensor imaging (DTI) to assess tracts, fMRI (see Discussion and Comments)

9.1   Discussion and Comments

Horizontal gaze palsy with progressive scoliosis (HGPPS) is an autosomal recessive disorder characterised by congenital absence of horizontal gaze, progressive scoliosis developing in childhood (◘ Fig. 9.1) and failure of the corticospinal and somatosensory tracts to decussate (◘ Fig. 9.4) [1, 2]. It results from a mutation in the axon guidance molecule ROBO3 [2].

There is an absence of the abducens nuclei (◘ Fig. 9.3) which coordinates the abducens nerve and the contralateral oculomotor nerve for smooth horizontal gaze. The pons and medulla oblongata show reduced volume (◘ Fig. 9.2) [1, 2].

Several pathogeneses of the scoliosis have been suggested and true aetiology remains a subject of debate. The most commonly accepted explanation is a primary neurological dysfunction.

The descending corticospinal and ascending sensory tracts in the affected individuals fail to cross the midline of the medulla in early development [1, 2].

Other causes of scoliosis must be excluded, such as congenital malformations of the spine and tumours. Neurofibromatosis can affect the entire central nervous system and cause nerve palsies.

HGPPS is one of several genetic disorders of eye control that are believed to result from cranial nuclei maldevelopment, the most closely related to HGPPS being Duane and Moebius syndrome. Abnormal development of the abducens nucleus plays a crucial role in the pathogenesis of all these entities [2].

Imaging findings (discussed above) are pathognomonic. Advanced imaging such as DTI and fMRI reveals only ipsilaterally ascending and descending connectivities and normal interhemispheric connections in the corpus callosum and ipsilateral activation in the primary motor cortex evoked by motor tasks [1].

References

1. Haller S, Wetzel SG, Lütschg J. Functional MRI, DTI and neurophysiology in horizontal gaze palsy with progressive scoliosis. Neuroradiology. 2008;50:453–9.
2. Rossi A, Catala M, Biancheri R, Di Comite R, Tortori-Donati PMR. MR Imaging of brain-stem hypoplasia in horizontal gaze palsy with progressive scoliosis. AJNR Am J Neuroradiol. 2004;25:1046–8.

Case 10

Nuno Ferreira Silva

© Springer International Publishing AG 2018
J. Xavier et al. (eds.), *Diagnostic and Therapeutic Neuroradiology*,
https://doi.org/10.1007/978-3-319-61140-2_10

A 33-day-old boy, without pre or perinatal relevant issues, aside from vacuum-assisted vaginal delivery, referred to the neuroradiology department for MRI evaluation (◘ Figs. 10.1, 10.2, 10.3, and 10.4) of a left cervical tumefaction, noted at about 5 days, seemingly enlarging and with concomitant neck movement restriction on the affected side. The child was otherwise normal and had no body temperature or routine laboratory test anomalies. Previously performed ultrasound was reported inconclusive.

? Questions

1. In which structure is the lesion centred and what is the pattern of involvement?
2. What other relevant findings stand out from the remaining neck structures/spaces?
3. What is the probable diagnosis and which plausible cause should be considered?

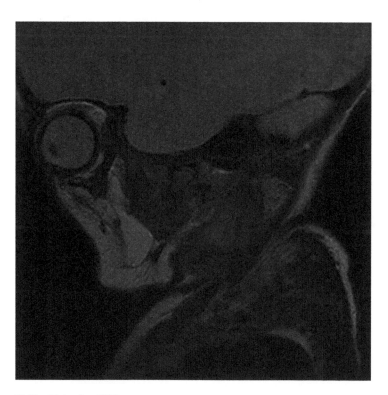

◘ **Fig. 10.1**   Sag T2WI

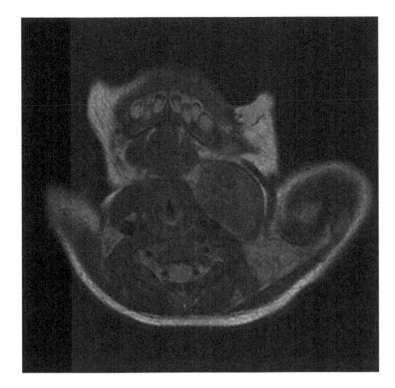

◘ **Fig. 10.2**   Axial T2WI

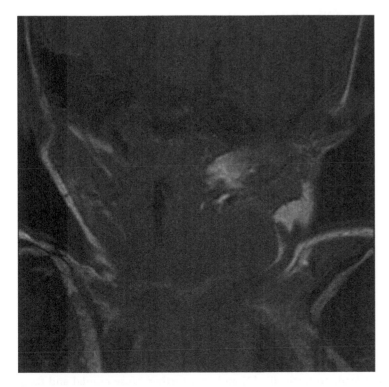

◘ **Fig. 10.3**   Coronal T1WI

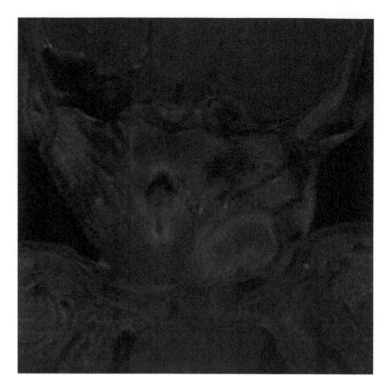

◘ **Fig. 10.4**   Post-contrast coronal T1WI

Diagnosis   Fibromatosis colli

✔ **Answers**
1. The lesion is centred in the left sternocleidomastoid muscle, involving it in a diffuse, fusiform and circumscribed pattern.
2. No other relevant findings are to be considered in the remaining neck spaces.
3. Clinical and imaging features are consistent with fibromatosis colli, dystocic delivery being the most likely cause.

10.1 Comments

Fibromatosis colli, also known as sternocleidomastoid tumour of infancy or congenital torticollis, refers to a fusiform enlargement of sternocleidomastoid muscle by benign fibrous tissue proliferation [2], not fully understood, but likely related to abnormal intrauterine foetal position or birth trauma. It is a relatively rare condition (0.4% of live births), slightly more frequent in males and mostly unilateral, with higher incidence on the right [1, 2, 3]. It typically presents between the second and fourth weeks after birth, affecting predominantly the distal two-thirds of the muscle [2]. In 14 to 20% of cases, it leads to torticollis [3] and may further cause cranial and facial dysmorphisms, as well as postural changes. However, it usually has a benign course, with sudden increase in size of the mass, stabilised within a few months and then gradually diminishing, with spontaneous resolution in 4 to 8 months.

The diagnosis is based upon clinical history, type of onset and progression profile, usually combined with ultrasonography evaluation. Equivocal cases may further require MRI investigation, namely, to discard other congenital lesions, infection, benign neoplasms and malignant conditions. Typical findings are diffuse, fusiform enlargement of the muscle, with variable echogenicity and signal intensity, and extensive contrast enhancement, tending to preserve fibre orientation.

Treatment is conservative, although surgery takes place in up to 10% of cases [2]. More recently, botulinum toxin type A administration has further decreased the need for invasive procedures in refractory cases [1, 2].

References

1. Tempark T, et al. Fibromatosis colli, overlooked cause of neonatal torticollis: a case report. Int J Pediatr Otorhinolarynglol Extra. 2012;7:15–7.
2. Khalid S, et al. Fibromatosis colli: a case report. Oman Med J. 2012;27(6):e011.
3. Adamoli P, et al. Rapid spontaneous resolution of fibromatosis colli in a 3-week-old girl. Case Rep Otolaryngol. 2014;2014:264940.

Inflammatory Diseases

Contents

Case 11

Bruno Moreira

© Springer International Publishing AG 2018
J. Xavier et al. (eds.), *Diagnostic and Therapeutic Neuroradiology*,
https://doi.org/10.1007/978-3-319-61140-2_11

A 4-year-old boy. A 3-month history of diabetes insipidus (⬛ Figs. 11.1, 11.2, 11.3, and 11.4).

❓ Questions

1. Which findings justify the history of diabetes insipidus?
2. What would be your differentials concerning the images of the sellar/suprasellar region?
3. Are there any additional findings that can narrow your differentials list?

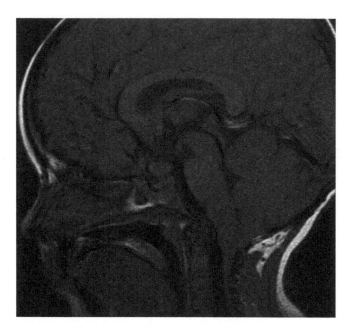

⬛ Fig. 11.1   Sag T1WI

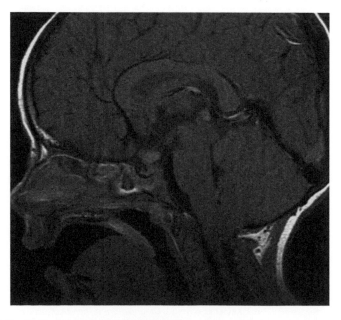

⬛ Fig. 11.2   Sag contrast-enhanced T1WI

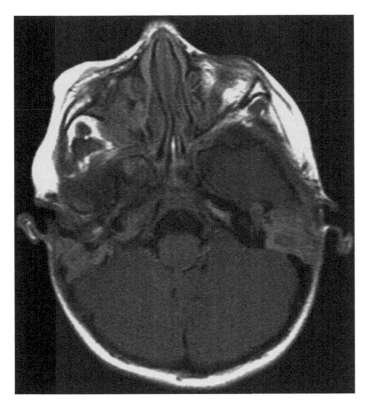

■ Fig. 11.3   Ax contrast-enhanced T1WI

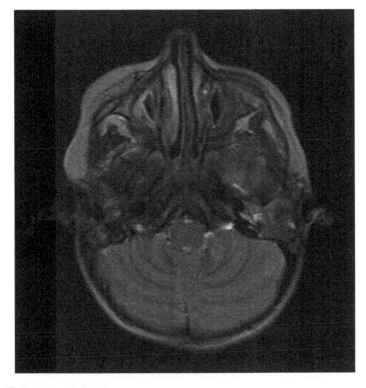

■ Fig. 11.4   Ax T2WI

Diagnosis   Langerhans cell histiocytosis (LCH)

✅ **Answers to Questions**

1. There is a hypothalamic/pituitary stalk lesion, centred in the median eminence, leading to diabetes insipidus (in the sagittal T1WI, we do not notice the posterior pituitary gland lobe bright spot, thought to be related to phospholipid or secretory granules contained in pituicytes).

2. The differentials should include inflammatory lesions (sarcoidosis, Wegener's granulomatosis, Churg-Strauss syndrome and lymphocytic hypophysitis) and neoplastic lesions (histiocytosis, granular cell tumour of the pituitary gland, germinoma, hypothalamic glioma, craniopharyngioma, lymphoma and metastasis).

3. Axial contrast-enhanced T1WI shows enhancing lesions in both mastoids, in the right retroantral fat pad and in the left pterygopalatine fossa. These findings narrow our differentials to histiocytosis, lymphoma and metastasis. The patient's age and the distribution of the lesions make histiocytosis much more likely.

11.1   Comments

Langerhans cell histiocytosis (LCH) is a rare disease of the dendritic cell system that may affect almost any organ. Recent studies indicate that LCH is caused by an uncontrolled clonal proliferation of dendritic cells with Langerhans cell characteristics [2].

It is currently regarded as a myeloid neoplasm (though it has long been controversial as to whether LCH is best considered a reactive process or a neoplasm), with a remarkably broad clinical spectrum, ranging from isolated skin or bone lesions to a disseminated disease that can involve nearly any organ. It is generally regarded as a sporadic disease which occurs predominantly in the paediatric population. The diagnosis of LCH is confirmed by immunohistochemistry (IHC) by demonstrating the presence of dendritic cell markers such as S100 protein, in addition to CD1a and langerin.

Prayer et al., in 2004, have classified the wide spectrum of intracranial findings in LCH patients into four major groups according to their anatomic topography and signal-intensity pattern. Group 1 includes osseous lesions in the craniofacial bones and/or skull base with or without soft tissue extension. Group 2 is an intracranial and extra-axial disease in the hypothalamic-pituitary region, meninges and other circumventricular organs, including the pineal gland, choroid plexus and ependyma. Group 3 is intra-axial parenchymal disease in the grey matter or white matter, with a striking symmetry of the lesions and a clear predominance of a neurodegenerative pattern in the cerebellum and basal ganglia. Group 4 is localized or diffuse atrophy [1].

No consensus exists for the optimal therapy for LCH, particularly in the case of multisystem organ disease. Nevertheless, patients with central nervous system involvement require therapy directed at their CNS lesions. Treatment options include chemotherapy that crosses the blood-brain barrier, resection, radiation therapy or a combination of these. These options have not been compared directly in a prospective trial.

References

1. Prayer D, et al. MR imaging presentation of intracranial disease associated with Langerhans cell Histiocytosis. Am J Neuroradiol. 2004;25:880–91.
2. Grois N, et al. Neuropathology of CNS disease in Langerhans cell histiocytosis. Brain. 2005;128:829–38.

Case 12

Sofia Pina

© Springer International Publishing AG 2018
J. Xavier et al. (eds.), *Diagnostic and Therapeutic Neuroradiology*,
https://doi.org/10.1007/978-3-319-61140-2_12

A 26-year-old man with focal seizures of the right hand for 1 week (◘ Figs. 12.1, 12.2, 12.3 and 12.4).

Follow up at 15 days. Clinical impairment with additional neurological deficits (◘ Figs. 12.5 and 12.6).

❓ Questions

1. Describe the imaging findings.
2. Point out the differential diagnoses.

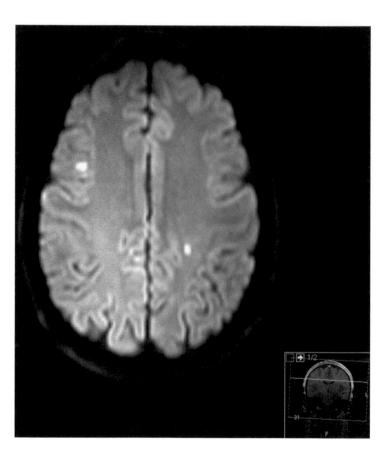

◘ Fig. 12.1   Axial DWI

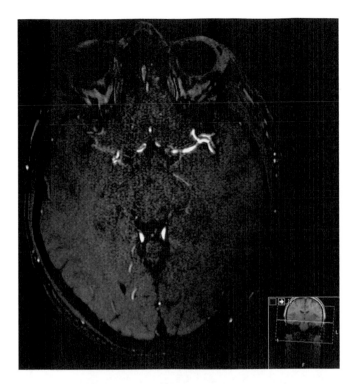

☐ **Fig. 12.2**   3D TOF

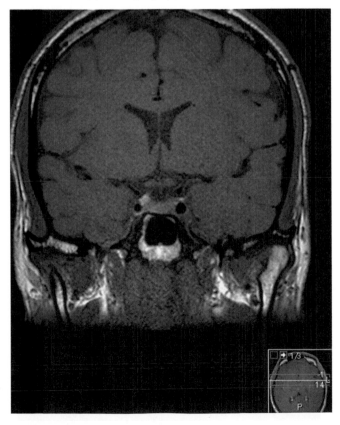

☐ **Fig. 12.3**   Coronal T1 WI without gadolinium

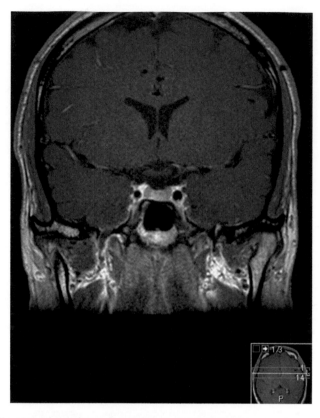

Fig. 12.4 Coronal T1 with gadolinium vessel wall imaging

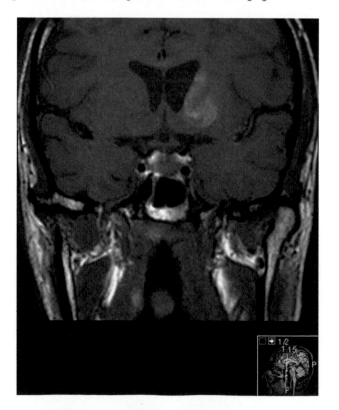

Fig. 12.5 Follow up coronal T1 WI

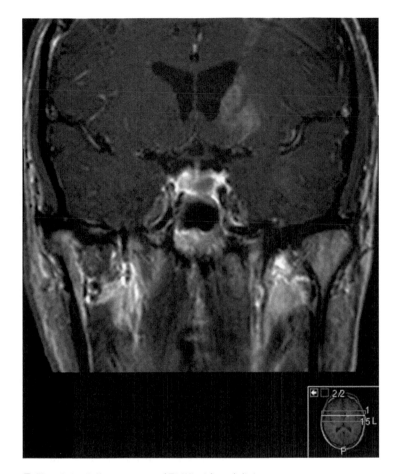

Fig. 12.6 Follow up coronal T1 WI with gadolinium

Diagnosis Primary angiitis of the central nervous system

✅ Answers
1. Multiple foci of restricted diffusion of water molecules (**Fig. 12.1**) suggest ischemia. Multiple focal stenoses of medium-sized intracranial arteries (**Fig. 12.2**). Enhancement of vessel walls confined to arterial constricted regions (**Fig. 12.4**) reveals inflammation. Between imaging studies, this patient developed new areas of infarction and new areas of concentric enhancement of arterial walls (**Fig. 12.5 and 12.6**).
2. Reversible cerebral vasoconstriction syndromes, systemic vasculitis, infection, atherosclerosis, emboli, intravascular lymphoma, Moyamoya disease, and amyloid angiopathy.

12.1 Comments

Central nervous system (CNS) vasculitis refers to a broad spectrum of diseases that result in inflammation and destruction of the blood vessels of the brain, spinal cord, and meninges. Primary angiitis of the CNS (PACNS) refers to vasculitis that is confined to the CNS and is a rare disease of unknown aetiology. Secondary CNS vasculitis is considered when this occurs in the context of a systemic inflammatory disease, such as a systemic vasculitis or systemic lupus erythematosus (SLE), or an infectious process such as varicella zoster virus [1].

PACNS predominantly affects small- and medium-sized arteries of the brain parenchyma, spinal cord, and leptomeninges, causing the vessels to become narrowed, occluded, and thrombosed, resulting in tissue ischemia and necrosis of the territories of the involved vessels and resulting in symptoms and signs of CNS dysfunction. It is defined by inflammation of the cerebral vasculature without angiitis in other organs. PACNS is a rare disease, the cause of which is unknown. There is a 2:1 male predominance and the median age at diagnosis is 50 years [1, 2].

The diagnosis of PACNS is challenging, as the symptoms are generally nonspecific and there is no specific diagnostic test, being a diagnosis of exclusion, the differential diagnoses including the reversible cerebral vasoconstriction syndromes and systemic vasculitis involving the brain such as Behçet's syndrome, polyarteritis nodosa, granulomatous disorder, systemic rheumatic diseases, antiphospholipid syndrome, infection, atherosclerosis, emboli, CADASIL, intravascular lymphoma, MELAS, Moyamoya disease, and amyloid angiopathy [1, 2, 3].

PACNS should be suspected when more often recurrent strokes occur in young patients with no identifiable cardiovascular or hypercoagulable risk factors; in the development of cognitive dysfunction with or without headaches; in recurrent or persistent focal neurological symptoms; and in abnormal cerebrovascular imaging obtained in the setting of an unexplained neurological deficit, or unexplained spinal cord dysfunction, not associated with systemic disease or any other process [1, 2, 3].

The CSF is abnormal in 80 to 90 percent of patients with pathologically documented disease. CSF findings are nonspecific but most commonly include an elevated CSF protein and a modest lymphocytic pleocytosis [1, 2].

MRI of the brain commonly shows multiple infarcts in multiple vascular territories, and vasculopathy is shown in MRA, CTA, or conventional angiography studies [1, 3].

Conventional angiography has poor specificity and low sensitivity. Brain biopsy is the gold standard but also with low sensitivity, and there should be a multidisciplinary discussion weighing risks and benefits [1, 2, 3].

High-resolution MRI with gadolinium allows the study of vessel walls in an active inflammatory phase, showing smooth, concentric wall enhancement and thickening. This pattern of the vessel wall has been proved to be remarkably different for CNS vasculitis and reversible cerebral vasoconstriction syndrome at initial imaging and at follow-up [3].

Treatment for the initial therapy of suspected PACNS with empiric glucocorticoids may be appropriate while the full workup is completed. Immunosuppressive therapy has been associated with success in central nervous system vasculitis [1, 2].

The response to treatment is monitored by periodic reassessment of symptoms, neurological findings, and neuroimaging abnormalities.

References

1. Hajj-Ali RA, Calabrese LH. Diagnosis and classification of central nervous system vasculitis. J Autoimmun. 2014;48-49:149.
2. Salvarani C, Brown RD Jr, Christianson TJ, et al. Adult primary central nervous system vasculitis treatment and course: analysis of one hundred sixty-three patients. Arthritis Rheumatol. 2015;67:1637.
3. Obusez EC, Hui F, Hajj-Ali RA, Cerejo R, Calabrese LH, Hammad T, et al. Vessel wall imaging: spatial and temporal patterns of reversible cerebral vasoconstriction syndrome and central nervous system vasculitis. AJNR Am J Neuroradiol. 2014;35(8):1527–32.

Case 13

Tiago Rodrigues

© Springer International Publishing AG 2018
J. Xavier et al. (eds.), *Diagnostic and Therapeutic Neuroradiology*,
https://doi.org/10.1007/978-3-319-61140-2_13

A 5-year-old boy with diabetes insipidus, diagnosed at the age of 3. There were no neurological signs or symptoms.

❓ Questions
1. What do the cerebellar signal changes reflect?
2. What is the differential diagnosis for the cerebellar signal abnormalities?
3. What other central nervous system lesions might be found in this disease?

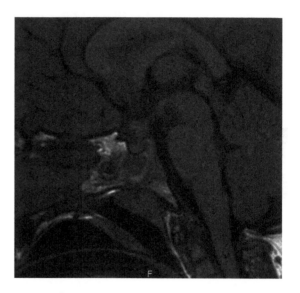

◘ **Fig. 13.1** Sagital T1-WI

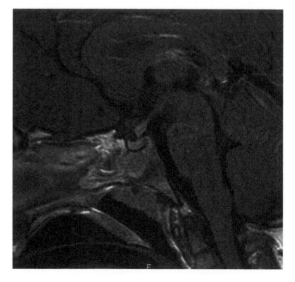

◘ **Fig. 13.2** Post contrast sagital T1-WI

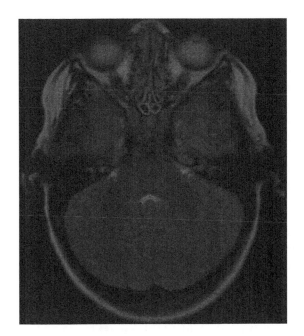

Fig. 13.3 Axial T2-WI, initial MRI

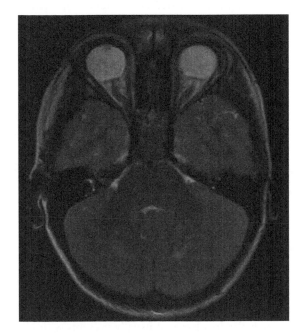

Fig. 13.4 Axial T2-WI, follow-up MRI

Diagnosis Neurodegenerative Langerhans cell histiocytosis (ND-LCH) (have you paid attention to ▶ Chap. 11?)

✓ **Answers**
1. Neurodegenerative changes with neuron loss, axonal degeneration and T-cell inflammation
2. Acute disseminated encephalomyelitis, metabolic/degenerative disorders, toxic demyelination, paraneoplastic encephalitis, haemophagocytic lymphohistiocytosis
3. Granulomas in the extra-axial space, in the brain parenchyma or in the spinal cord and bone lesions

13.1 Captions

High-resolution sagittal T1-WI (◘ Fig. 13.1) and sagittal postcontrast T1-WI (◘ Fig. 13.2) images revealed absence of the T1 neurohypophysis high signal and nodular thickening and enhancement of the pituitary stalk.

Axial T2-WI at the initial MRI scan (◘ Fig. 13.3) showed bilateral symmetric high signal abnormalities in the dentate nuclei and in the surrounding white matter. On the follow-up MRI (6 months later), there was progression of the T2 high signal cerebellar changes (◘ Fig. 13.4).

13.2 Comments

Central nervous system (CNS) involvement occurs in approximately 23–35% of the children with Langerhans cell histiocytosis (LCH) and, from the imaging standpoint, can be divided into space-occupying lesions (◘ Figs. 13.1 and 13.2) and neurodegenerative changes (known as "neurodegenerative Langerhans cell histiocytosis" (ND-LCH)).

ND-LCH can occur in 4–10% of the paediatric LCH and represent diffuse inflammatory brain damage with consequent neuronal, axonal and myelin destruction leading to atrophy. Most often, there are bilateral symmetric lesions in the cerebellum, the basal ganglia and/or the brainstem, with variable signal intensity on MR imaging depending on the site and stage of the disease. In the initial inflammatory phase, sharply demarcated enhancement foci might be seen. Cerebellar involvement usually presents with bilateral T2 hyperintense lesions in the dentate nuclei and the deep cerebellar white matter (◘ Fig. 13.3). Regarding basal ganglia changes, there is more commonly bilateral and symmetric T1 hyperintensity in the pallidum [1, 2].

The neurodegenerative MRI changes are irreversible and tend to be slowly progressive (◘ Fig. 13.4), but clinical manifestations are highly variable, ranging from absence of neurological deficits to a severe clinical picture, including ataxia, motor spasticity, dysarthria, dysphagia, intellectual disability or severe psychiatric disease [1].

References

1. Prosch H, et al. Long-term MR imaging course of neurodegenerative Langerhans cell Histiocytosis. AJNR. 2007;28:1022–8.
2. Schmidt S, et al. Extraosseous Langerhans cell Histiocytosis in children. Radiographics. 2008;28(3):707–26.

Case 14

Tiago Rodrigues

© Springer International Publishing AG 2018
J. Xavier et al. (eds.), *Diagnostic and Therapeutic Neuroradiology*,
https://doi.org/10.1007/978-3-319-61140-2_14

A 50-year-old female patient with a history of morning stiffness and arthralgias for 20 years presented with headaches, fever, dysphasia and right hemiparesis. The CSF analysis revealed mononuclear pleocytosis (190cells/mm^3), and on the serological evaluation, there was an elevation of rheumatoid factor and anticitrulline antibodies.

? **Questions**
1. What are the causes of FLAIR subarachnoid space hyperintensity?
2. What are the differential diagnoses in this case?
3. What other CNS lesions might be associated with this disease?

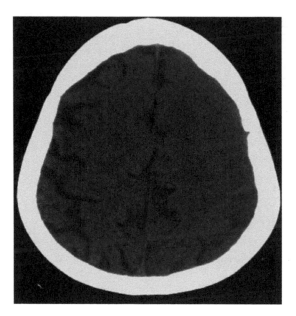

▪ Fig. 14.1   Initial CT scan T1-WI

14

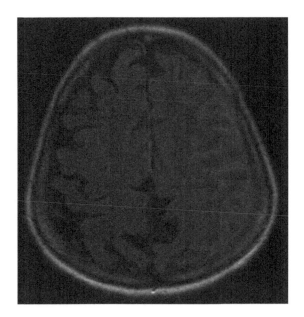

■ Fig. 14.2　Axial T1-WI

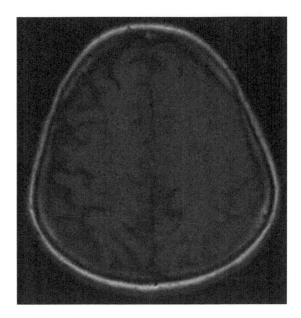

■ Fig. 14.3　Axial T2 FLAIR image

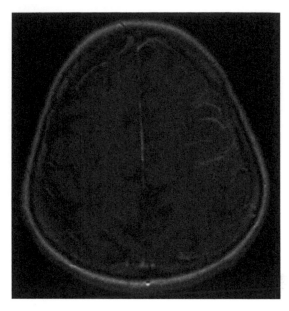

⊡ Fig. 14.4   Post contrast axial T1-WI

Diagnosis   Rheumatoid meningitis

✅ **Answers**
1. Subarachnoid haemorrhage, meningitis, meningeal carcinomatosis, leptomeningeal melanosis, acute stroke (slow flow), Moyamoya disease, fat-containing lesions, supplemental oxygen and artefacts (vascular pulsation artefact, CSF flow artefact, motion artefact)
2. Inflammatory/infectious meningitis and leptomeningeal carcinomatosis
3. Vasculitis and rheumatoid nodules

14.1 Comments

Central nervous system (CNS) involvement is a rare but serious complication of rheumatoid arthritis. It can occur as pachymeningitis or leptomeningitis, vasculitis (related to a lymphoplasmacytic infiltrate in the vessel walls) or rheumatoid nodules.

Rheumatoid meningitis is one of the most serious complications of rheumatoid arthritis, and its diagnosis is critical since the disease can be treated with immunosuppressants. The imaging findings are nonspecific and common to other forms of meningitis and to leptomeningeal carcinomatosis. The inflammatory process that fills the subarachnoid space in rheumatoid arthritis might exhibit isodensity on CT (⊡ Fig. 14.1), T1 and T2 isointensity (⊡ Fig. 14.2), FLAIR hyperintensity (⊡ Fig. 14.3), restricted diffusion on DWI and contrast enhancement (⊡ Fig. 14.4). The CSF study and even a brain biopsy can be nonspecific, pointing to an unspecified inflammatory process. Therefore, in cases in which the diagnosis of rheumatoid arthritis is not previously established (such as in this case), the serological findings are essential, namely, the elevation of rheumatoid factors and, more specifically, of anticitrulline antibodies. [1, 2]

References

1. Kim H, et al. A case of rheumatoid meningitis: pathologic and magnetic resonance imaging findings. Neurol Sci. 2011;32(6):1191–4.
2. Jones SE, et al. Rheumatoid meningitis: radiologic and pathologic correlation. Am J Roentgenol. 2006;186:1181–3.

Case 15

José Eduardo Alves

© Springer International Publishing AG 2018
J. Xavier et al. (eds.), *Diagnostic and Therapeutic Neuroradiology*,
https://doi.org/10.1007/978-3-319-61140-2_15

A 37-year-old male, with previous onset of bilateral hearing loss, vertigo, headaches, and progressive cognitive decline 2 years ago. Presents with sudden right hemiparesis and paresthesia. On the neurological examination, he was disoriented, with incoherent speech and attention deficit. There was mild right hemibody and face weakness and bilateral Babinski sign.

? Questions

1. What is the name of the characteristic callosal lesions depicted in B and D?
2. Based on the clinical picture and on the MRI findings, what is the diagnosis?
3. What other organ should be thoroughly assessed to look for disease involvement?

15

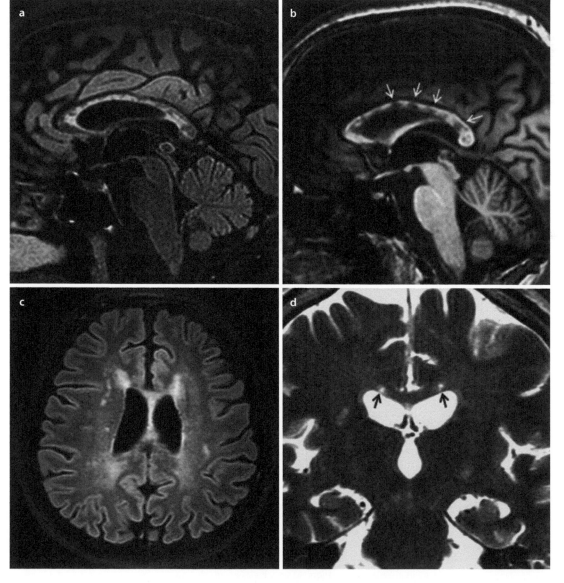

▫ Fig. 15.1   MRI **a** sagittal and **c** axial T2 FLAIR, **b** sagittal T1 3D and **d** coronal T2 TSE

Diagnosis   Susac's syndrome

 Answers
1. Callosal *holes* (B) and *snowballs* (D)
2. Susac's syndrome
3. The eyes

15.1   Comments

Susac's syndrome is an autoimmune endotheliopathy, most commonly affecting women between the third and fourth decades. Clinically, it's characterized by encephalopathy, multifocal bilateral scotomas (due to branch retinal artery occlusions), and sensorineural hearing loss (caused by obstruction of small vessels supplying cochlea). Neurological involvement is usually self-limited (1 to 3 years) and diverse, including cognitive dysfunction, behavioral problems, gait disturbances, dysarthria, and headaches.

Brain MRI plays an essential role in pointing toward the diagnosis, especially in cases where the clinical triad is not present. The most typical feature is the presence of multiple microinfarcts in the central portion of the corpus callosum – *snowballs* on T2-weighted images (◘ Fig. 15.1d) – that, when cavitated, become the almost pathognomonic T1-weighted callosal *holes* (◘ Fig. 15.1b). Callosal linear microinfarcts show *icicle* and *spoke* configurations (◘ Fig. 15.1a), and the presence of multiple infarcts in the posterior limbs of the internal capsules gives origin to a *string of pearls* image, also typical of this entity [1].

However, brain involvement is usually widespread, including multiple supratentorial periventricular and subcortical white matter lesions (◘ Fig. 15.1c), deep gray matter, cerebellum, and brainstem involvement. In the acute stage, lesions may show contrast enhancement, which occasionally extends to the leptomeninges [2].

References

1. Seghers A, et al. Characteristic callosal involvement in Susac's syndrome. Acta Neurol Belg. 2015;115(3):395–6.
2. Susac J, et al. MRI findings in Susac's syndrome. Neurology. 2003;61:1783–7.

Infectious Diseases

Contents

Case 16

Daniela Jardim Pereira and Paula Gouveia

© Springer International Publishing AG 2018
J. Xavier et al. (eds.), *Diagnostic and Therapeutic Neuroradiology*,
https://doi.org/10.1007/978-3-319-61140-2_16

A 2-year-old boy, with a 1-day history of fever, nasal congestion and coughing, was admitted to the emergency department due to altered mental state. A few hours later, he developed right hemiparesis and left oculomotor nerve palsy, followed by neurological deterioration, needing intubation and admission to the intensive care unit. Head CT on day 1 showed bilateral thalamic hypodensities. MRI was performed on day 4 after admission (◘ Fig. 16.1).

? Questions
1. What are the main structures involved?
2. Which three different components can we distinguish in thalamic lesions?
3. Point out five radiological differential diagnoses.

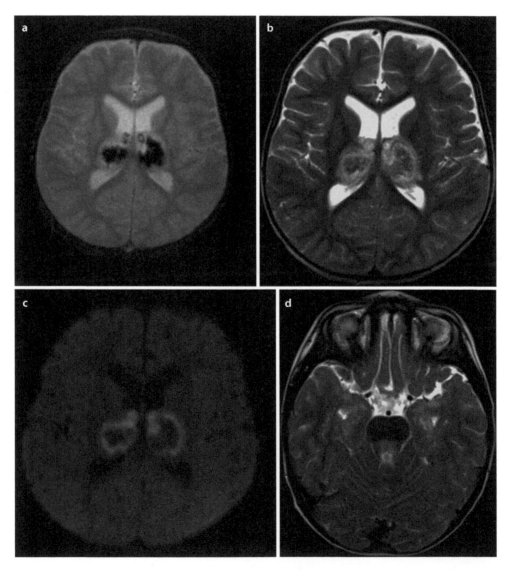

◘ **Fig. 16.1**   MRI axial T2* **a**, T2-weighted image **b** and diffusion-weighted image **c**, showing bilateral thalamic enlargement with low sign on T2WI and T2* centrally, surrounded by a thin halo of restricted diffusion and high sign on T2 at the periphery. Additionally, we identify bilateral and symmetrical diffuse T2 hyperintensity on the pontine tegmentum and hippocampus **d**

Diagnosis Acute necrotizing encephalopathy (ANE) caused by H1N1.

✅ Answers to Questions

1. Bilateral and symmetrical involvement of the thalamus, upper brainstem tegmentum and hippocampus. There were also small-scattered foci on cingulate and frontal cortex bilaterally, including the left precentral gyrus (not shown).
2. A haemorrhagic necrotic centre, surrounded by cytotoxic oedema and an outside portion of vasogenic oedema, in a typical «tricolour pattern» or target-like appearance.
3. Arterial or venous infarct (excluded by MR angiography), Leigh syndrome, severe hypoxia, Wernicke's encephalopathy and acute disseminated encephalopathy (excluded by the clinical history and laboratory findings).

16.1 Comments

ANE is a parainfectious disease triggered by a viral infection, including novel influenza A (H1N1) among other possible agents. The pathogenesis is still unclear, but the main hypotheses is that an amplified pro-inflammatory response with hypercytokinemia will lead to proteolysis of the blood-brain barrier and increase vessel wall permeability, explaining both the vasogenic and cytotoxic oedema and the haemorrhagic necrosis [1]. Lesions are bilaterally and quite symmetrically distributed, with the thalamus being affected in all patients [1, 2]. The upper brainstem tegmentum, cerebellum and white matter are also frequently involved. In rare cases, it may affect the meninges and spinal cord, which was excluded in our patient by MRI on day 7. There is no specific treatment for ANE and the mortality rate reaches 30%; however, early diagnosis with the establishment of supportive measures may improve the prognosis [3].

References

1. Wu X, Wu W, Pan W, Wu L, Liu K, Zhang HL. Acute necrotizing encephalopathy: an underrecognized clinicoradiologic disorder. Mediat Inflamm. 2015;2015:9–13. https://doi.org/10.1155/2015/792578
2. Ormitti F, Ventura E, Summa A, Picetti E, Crisi G. Acute necrotizing encephalopathy in a child during the 2009 influenza A(H1N1) pandemia: MR imaging in diagnosis and follow-up. Am J Neuroradiol. 2010;31(3):396–400. https://doi.org/10.3174/ajnr.A2058
3. Mariotti P, Iorio R, Frisullo G, Plantone D, Colantonio R, Tartaglione T, Valentini P. Acute necrotizing encephalopathy during novel influenza A (H1N1) virus infection. Ann Neurol. 2010;68(1):111–4. https://doi.org/10.1002/ana.21996

Case 17

Luís Cardoso and José Eduardo Alves

© Springer International Publishing AG 2018
J. Xavier et al. (eds.), *Diagnostic and Therapeutic Neuroradiology*,
https://doi.org/10.1007/978-3-319-61140-2_17

A 79-year-old female, demented patient, lives in a nursing facility; presented with incidental finding of space-occupying lesion on brain CT after a fall, neurological examination with anisocoria R > L and raised sedimentation rate in blood test, otherwise normal.

❓ Questions

1. What are the findings on these MR images?
2. What would be your differential diagnosis?
3. What other organs/structures could be involved by the same pathologic process and help increase diagnostic accuracy?

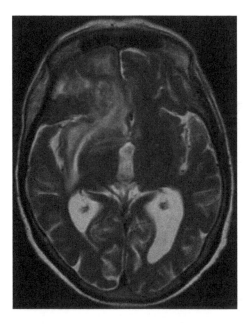

☐ **Fig. 17.1**   Axial T2

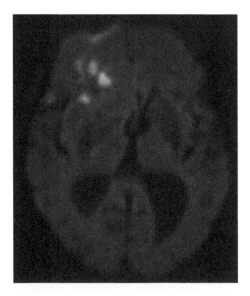

☐ **Fig. 17.2**   Axial DWI

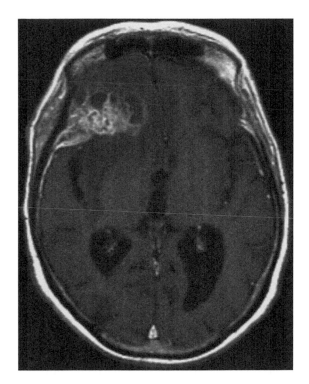

◘ **Fig. 17.3**   Axial T1 post gadolinium

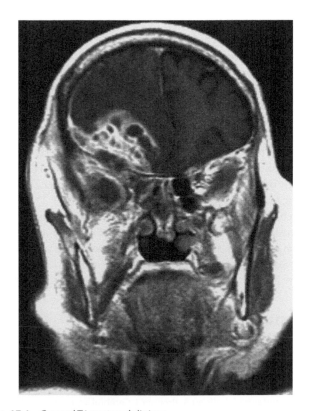

◘ **Fig. 17.4**   Coronal T1 post gadolinium

Diagnosis   Cerebral aspergillosis

✔ **Answers to Questions**

1. An extra- and intraparenchymal mass lesion, heterogeneous, with a dark T2 component and multiloculated appearance (◘ Fig. 17.1). Some loculated areas show reduced diffusion (◘ Fig. 17.2), and, after gadolinium, there is heterogeneous enhancement (partially with ring configuration) of the mass, as well as defuse enhancement of the dura (◘ Figs. 17.3 and 17.4).
2. Infectious process (pyogenic, tuberculosis, fungal) and aggressive neoplasm (glioblastoma, gliosarcoma, metastases).
3. Lungs and paranasal sinuses.

17.1 Comments

With the increasing prevalence of immunosuppressed patients, invasive aspergillosis of the central nervous system is becoming more frequent. Brain infection is frequently associated with pulmonary or paranasal sinus infections and reaches the brain through either hematogneous or direct spread [1, 2].

Aspergillus is angioinvasive, which is why it may lead to acute infarcts (septic emboli) and mycotic aneurysms, with an increased risk of subarachnoid bleed [1].

Symptoms of cerebral aspergillosis are nonspecific, including focal neurological deficits, seizures, cognitive changes and lethargy; fever may be present or absent.

On MRI, fungal infections may show characteristic peripheral low T2 and T2* sign. This is not associated with a significant haemorrhagic phenomenon but rather reflects the intermediate layers composed of a dense hyphal rim and peripheral inflammatory hypercellularity. These layers show contrast enhancement in 61% of the abscesses and are no longer believed to depend on the patient's immune status and the amount of inflammatory reaction [1].

A central intermediate signal on T2-weighted sequences may be present (corresponding to coagulative fungal necrosis at autopsy findings) and surrounded by a high hyperintense signal due to vasogenic oedema. Another feature that may be present is the characteristic target-like ADC signal lesion [2].

Cerebral fungal abscesses often display central areas of high signal intensity on DWI. This finding is associated with the restricted diffusion of water in the presence of proteinaceous fluid with coagulative necrosis. This last technique appears to be the most sensitive modality for early identification of cerebral aspergillosis [1].

References

1. Marzolf G, Sabou M, Lannes B, et al. Magnetic resonance imaging of cerebral Aspergillosis: imaging and pathological correlations. Zhang H, ed. PLoS One. 2016;11(4):e0152475. ▶ https://doi.org/10.1371/journal.pone.0152475.
2. Cox J, Murtagh FR, Wilfong A, Brenner J. Cerebral aspergillosis: MR imaging and histopathologic correlation. AJNR Am J Neuroradiol. 1992;13:1489–92.

Case 18

Gonçalo Basílio, André Rodrigues, and Lia Neto

© Springer International Publishing AG 2018
J. Xavier et al. (eds.), *Diagnostic and Therapeutic Neuroradiology*,
https://doi.org/10.1007/978-3-319-61140-2_18

A 38-year-old male patient presents with sudden onset of left eyelid oedema and left ocular pain which worsen with eye movements.

? Questions

1. What is the differential diagnosis of the first image?
2. What is the most common clinical presentation of the brain injuries in this pathology?
3. What is the most likely stage of the pathology?

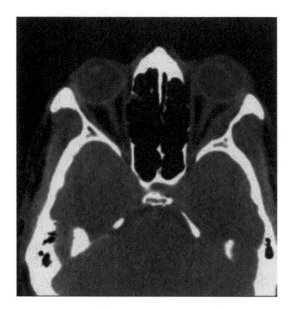

◘ Fig. 18.1   Axial CT – thickening of the left lateral rectus muscle

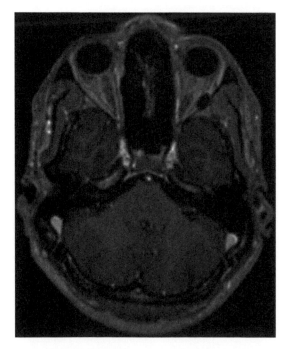

◘ Fig. 18.2   Axial T1 C+ – thickening of the left lateral rectus muscle with cystic hypointense lesion

18

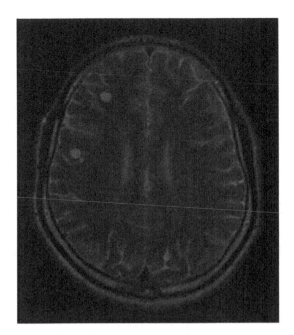

Fig. 18.3 Axial T2 – cystic lesions in the right frontal lobe, without surrounding oedema

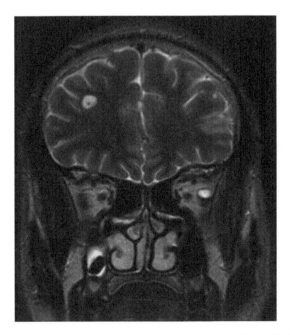

Fig. 18.4 Coronal T2 – cystic lesions in the right frontal lobe and left lateral rectus muscle, without surrounding oedema

Diagnosis Cysticercosis of the extraocular muscle and brain.

✅ **Answers to Questions**

  1. The first image (🔲 Fig. 18.1) shows a thickening of the left lateral rectus muscle, and the differential diagnosis includes Graves' disease, myositic form of idiopathic inflammation of

the orbit, arteriovenous fistula and malformations, orbital tumours and cysticercosis.
2. Seizures.
3. Vesicular stage as the cysts in the brain have a signal evolution similar to the CSF, with a dot sign visible that corresponds to the scolex (■ Figs. 18.3 and 18.4). There is no surrounding oedema in the parenchyma (■ Figs. 18.3 and 18.4). There is no significant enhancement of the cyst (■ Fig. 18.2).

18.1 Comments

Cysticercosis is found equally among both sexes and can be diagnosed at any age. It represents a heavy social burden in developing countries, reaching a 50 million world prevalence according to the Centers for Disease Control. The neurological manifestations can lead to death in about 15% of all patients. Cysticercosis usually affects highly vascularized tissues such as the brain, the masticatory muscles, the tongue and the heart [2]. In the eye, the most common site for cysticercosis is the vitreous and subretinal spaces, followed by orbit and adnexal tissues[1]. The infection of the extraocular muscles can lead to restricted eye movements and inflammatory signs.

Imaging studies such as ultrasonography, CT scan and MRI can be helpful, especially when a cystic formation or calcification inside the muscle is documented [2].

Early treatment with oral albendazole and corticosteroids and cyst removal can be successful in restoring normal function [2].

References

1. Damani M, Mehta V, Nakwa B. Orbital cysticercosis: a case report. Saudi J Ophtalmol. 2012;26(4):457–8.
2. Angotti Neto H., Gonçalves AC, Moura FC, Monteiro ML; Extraocular muscle cysticercosis mimicking idiopathic orbital inflammation: case report. Arq. Bras. Oftalmol. 2007;70(3):537–9. São Paulo.

18

Case 19

José Eduardo Alves

© Springer International Publishing AG 2018
J. Xavier et al. (eds.), *Diagnostic and Therapeutic Neuroradiology*,
https://doi.org/10.1007/978-3-319-61140-2_19

A 31-day-old infant, born uneventfully at term, presented with poor feeding and insufficient weight gain. After admission, she had an episode of hyporeactivity, severe hypotonia, cyanosis and fixed gaze that lasted for a few minutes. She was afebrile and had no rash, petechiae or vesicular lesions. Complete blood count was normal. The cerebrospinal fluid had normal white blood cells and glucose levels and increased proteins.

❓ Questions

1. What is the most likely nature of the T1 hyperintensity in b?
2. What type of tissue is mainly involved in c and d?
3. What would be your differential diagnosis?

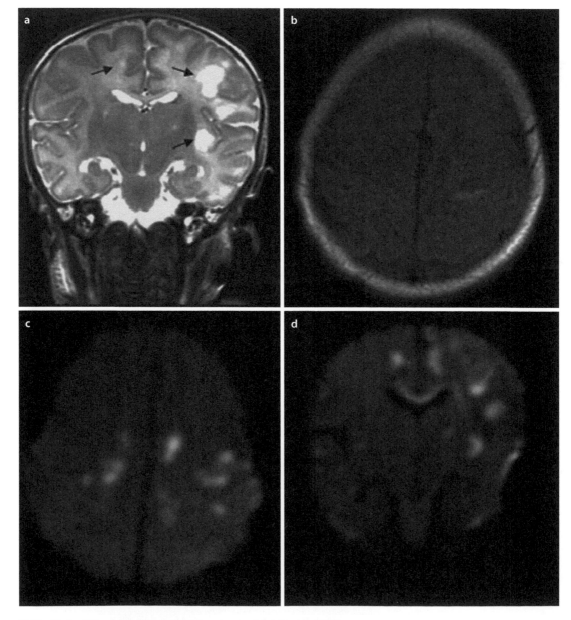

⬛ **Fig. 19.1**   MRI **a** coronal T2, **b** axial T1 and **c, d** axial and coronal DWI

19

Diagnosis   Enterovirus 71 encephalitis

✅ **Answers**
1. Haemorrhagic
2. White matter
3. Infectious encephalitis or postinfectious autoimmune encephalitis

19.1 Comments

Enterovirus (EV) and parechovirus infections are common in infants, mostly during summer and autumn. Although rare, neurological complications of EV 71 infection are well known, including meningitis, brainstem encephalitis and acute flaccid paralysis. Involvement of the posterior portions of the medulla oblongata and pons is a characteristic finding, not present in our patient.

In the literature, there are scarce descriptions of severe white matter damage associated with neonatal EV encephalitis. The pathogenesis of white matter damage is unclear and may be attributable to inflammatory cytokines generated during the infectious process or to direct viral invasion [1].

On MRI, white matter lesions are better detected on DWI, due to reduced diffusion in the acute stage (◼ Fig. 19.1c, d), while T1- and T2-weighted sequences might depict petechial haemorrhages (◼ Fig. 19.1a, b).

The extent of the diffusion changes often suggests a more adverse outcome than in reality, so the correlation between severity of imaging abnormalities and neurodevelopmental outcome is not well established [2].

References

1. Ong KC, Wong KT. Understanding enterovirus 71 neuropathogenesis and its impact on other neurotropic enteroviruses. Brain Pathol. 2015;25:614–24.
2. Verboon-Maciolek MA, et al. White matter damage in neonatal enterovirus meningoencephalitis. Neurology. 2006;66:1267–9.

Case 20

Alexandra C. Lopes and Daniel Dias

© Springer International Publishing AG 2018
J. Xavier et al. (eds.), *Diagnostic and Therapeutic Neuroradiology*,
https://doi.org/10.1007/978-3-319-61140-2_20

Clinical Information 11-year-old female presenting with a subacute (3 weeks) febrile syndrome, occipital and right frontoparietal headache, weight loss and right torticollis. Laboratory tests: erythrocyte sedimentation rate (ESR) and C-reactive protein (CRP) levels elevated.

❓ Questions

1. Name the findings.
2. What is the diagnosis and possible associated complications?
3. What are the possible causes?

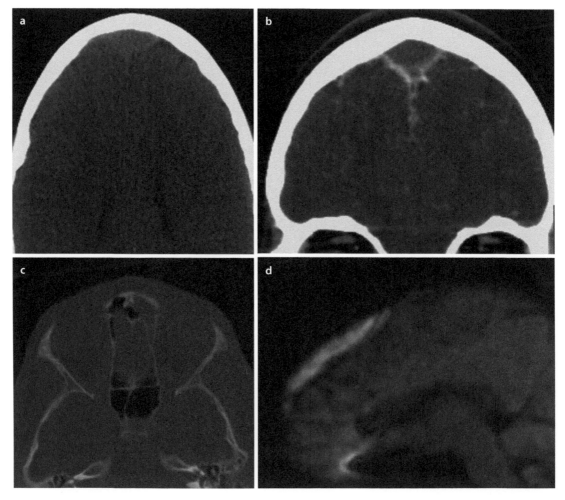

◘ Fig. 20.1 **a** Non-contrast head CT, axial view; **b** contrast-enhanced head CT, coronal reconstruction; **c** paranasal CT, axial view; **d** sagittal diffusion-weighted cerebral images

20

Diagnosis   Cerebral epidural empyema

✅ **Answers**

1. Extra-axial epidural frontal midline collection (◙ Fig. 20.1a, b) with reduced water diffusion (◙ Fig. 20.1d); left frontal sinus soft tissue opacification – inflammatory process (◙ Fig. 20.1c)
2. Intracranial epidural empyema; longitudinal superior sinus thrombosis (◙ Fig. 20.1b)
3. Direct extension of sinusitis or otitis media into the extracranial space; purulent meningitis

20.1 Comments

Sinogenic intracranial empyema is an uncommon complication of sinusitis [1] and a neurosurgical emergency [2]. It requires prompt diagnosis and treatment [1]. If not treated, it progresses rapidly and induces increased intracranial pressure with subsequent coma and death [2].

In a patient with sinusitis or otitis media, the infection is more likely to extend intracranially via the valveless diploic veins [1, 2]; it may also erode the facial bones causing osteomyelitis.

The clinical triad of fever, headache and altered mental status that is often reported in adults is not always present in paediatric patients. It is important to be aware of its variable clinical presentation and to highlight the relevance of laboratory tests and imagiologic findings.

Imaging studies should be performed immediately when this diagnosis is suspected [1], contrast-enhanced computed tomography (CECT) being the first-line choice; magnetic resonance imaging (MRI) with gadolinium is considered the gold standard for diagnosing any sinogenic intracranial complication [1], namely, empyema and its potential complications, such as venous sinus thrombosis [2].

In our case, the clinical presentation and the unawareness of sinusitis did not immediately raise the clinical suspicion of intracranial empyema. However, laboratory test results and the patient's symptoms justified additional imaging investigation, and the diagnosis was achieved; CECT and MRI also displayed frontal sinus signs of inflammation and partial thrombosis of the superior longitudinal sinus.

References

1. Adame N, Hedlund G, Byington CL. Sinogenic intracranial empyema in children. Pediatrics. 2005;116(3):e461–7.
2. Weingarten K, Zimmerman RD, Becker RD, Heier LA, Haimes AB, MDF D. Subdural and epidural empyemas: MR imaging. AJNR. 1989;10:81–7. 0195-6108/89/1001-0081.

Case 21

Sofia Pina, José Pedro Rocha Pereira, Ricardo Taipa, and Manuel Melo Pires

© Springer International Publishing AG 2018
J. Xavier et al. (eds.), *Diagnostic and Therapeutic Neuroradiology*,
https://doi.org/10.1007/978-3-319-61140-2_21

A 60-year-old man presents with apathy for 3 months and progressive installation of language disorder, right hemianopia, and right motor deficit (⬛ Figs. 21.1, 21.2, 21.3, 21.4, and 21.5).

❓ **Questions**
  1. What are the findings?
  2. What are the differential diagnoses based on imaging?
  3. Name other pathologies frequently associated with this entity.

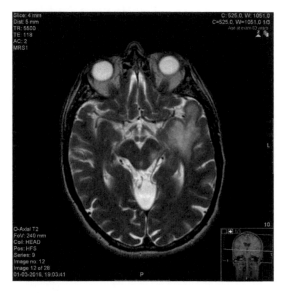

⬛ **Fig. 21.1**   Axial T2WI

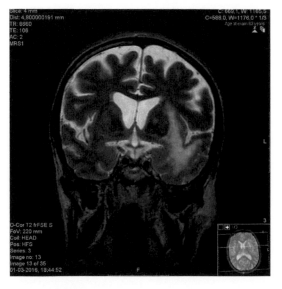

⬛ **Fig. 21.2**   Coronal T2WI

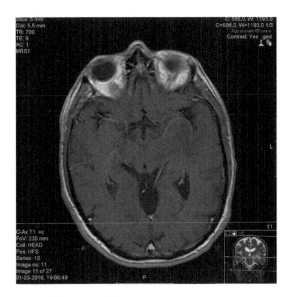

Fig. 21.3 Axial T1 with Gadolinium

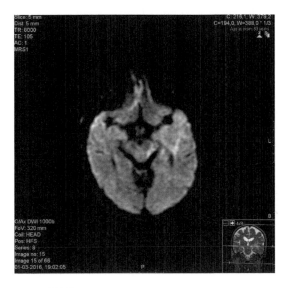

Fig. 21.4 Axial DWI

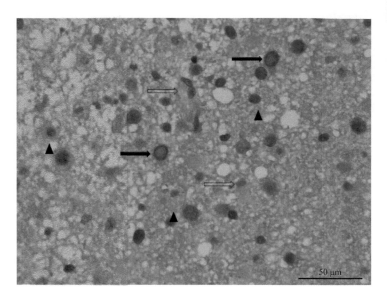

◘ Fig. 21.5 Hematoxylin and eosin staining scale bar 50 μm

Diagnosis   Progressive multifocal leukoencephalopathy (PML)

✔ Answers

1. Left temporal lobe subcortical white matter signal change extending into the external capsule and left midbrain, hypointense on T1WI, hyperintense on T2WI with microcystic appearance, and hyperintense DWI WI at deep periphery, without enhancement (◘ Figs. 21.1 – 4). Neuropathology H&E (◘ Fig. 21.5), scale bar 50 μm reveals severe demyelinating lesion with macrophages (arrow heads), atypical astrocytes (white arrows), and PML-intranuclear inclusions (black arrows).
2. Infiltrative tumour, lymphoma, infarct, vasculitis, PRES, and granulomatous disease.
3. HIV (in the present case, the diagnosis of AIDS was made days after the MR scanning), haematological disorders, solid organ malignancies, granulomatous, inflammatory diseases (e.g. patients with multiple sclerosis under natalizumab), and organ transplant recipients.

21.1   Comments

Progressive multifocal leukoencephalopathy (PML) is a severe demyelinating disease of the central nervous system that is caused by reactivation of the polyomavirus JC (JC virus) that occurs almost exclusively in immunosuppressed individuals [1, 2, 3].

PML was recognised as a major opportunistic infection associated with AIDS in adults, with a prevalence of 1–5%. Since the widespread use of HAART, the incidence of PML in patients with HIV infection has decreased. In addition, PML may improve or stabilise with potent antiretroviral therapy, leading to prolonged survival [2].

21

Outside of HIV infection, PML occurs in rare cases of patients with lymphoproliferative and myeloproliferative diseases, solid organ malignancies, granulomatous and inflammatory diseases, and organ transplant recipients. Rare cases of PML have been reported in patients treated with the immunomodulatory medication natalizumab. Most patients with HIV infection and PML are profoundly immunosuppressed with CD4-positive T-cell counts <200 per mm^3 [2].

The disease course of PML is usually progressive and fatal. The median survival of patients without HIV infection is only a few months, being longer in those under highly active antiretroviral therapy; survivors are often being left with severe neurological sequelae.

PML usually manifests with subacute neurological deficits including altered mental status, motor deficits (hemiparesis or monoparesis), limb ataxia, gait ataxia, and visual symptoms such as hemianopsia and diplopia [1, 2, 3].

The typical neuroimaging pattern shows multifocal areas of white matter demyelination that do not conform to cerebrovascular territories and exhibit neither mass effect nor contrast enhancement, although atypical enhancing lesions have been described, some representing PML-IRIS in the appropriate setting of new symptomatology after the introduction of HAART. PML lesions can appear as hypodense patchy or confluent white matter regions on CT and as areas of decreased signal on T1-weighted images, increased signal on T2-weighted and fluid-attenuated inversion recovery (FLAIR) sequences and hyperintense on diffusion-weighted sequences on MRI [1, 3].

Preferentially involving periventricular areas and the subcortical white matter, it may involve the corpus callosum, brainstem, pyramidal tracts, and cerebellum, and less frequently, the deep grey structures [1, 2, 3].

Diagnostic certainty is achieved by the finding of JC virus DNA in the cerebrospinal fluid (CSF) using polymerase chain reaction (PCR). However, brain biopsy remains the gold standard technique for the diagnosis. Neuropathology reveals demyelination, mainly involving the subcortical white matter, but also the grey matter, with JC virus infecting cortical neurons, bizarre astrocytes, and enlarged oligodendroglial nuclei. The presence of JC virus-infected glial or cortical cells should be confirmed by immunohistochemistry for polyomavirus proteins or in situ hybridisation for JC virus DNA [1, 2, 3].

References

1. Bag AK, Curé JK, Chapman PR, Roberson GH, Shah R. JC virus infection of the brain. AJNR Am J Neuroradiol. 2010;31(9):1564–76. https://doi.org/10.3174/ajnr.A2035. Epub 2010 Mar 18.
2. Engsig FN, Hansen AB, Omland LH, et al. Incidence, clinical presentation, and outcome of progressive multifocal leukoencephalopathy in HIV-infected patients during the highly active antiretroviral therapy era: a nationwide cohort study. J Infect Dis. 2009;199:77.
3. Sahraian MA, Radue EW, Eshaghi A, et al. Progressive multifocal leukoencephalopathy: a review of the neuroimaging features and differential diagnosis. Eur J Neurol. 2012;19:1060.

Case 22

Fidel Bastos, João Comba, and Teresa Bernardo

© Springer International Publishing AG 2018
J. Xavier et al. (eds.), *Diagnostic and Therapeutic Neuroradiology*,
https://doi.org/10.1007/978-3-319-61140-2_22

A 31-year-old black male with no history of smoking or alcoholism and negative results for HIV has suffered for approximately 8 months with intermittent lower back pain of rapidly progressive installation, associated with anorexia, weight loss and non-specific headache (◼ Figs. 22.1, 22.2, 22.3, and 22.4).

❓ Questions
1. What are the findings?
2. What are the differential diagnoses?

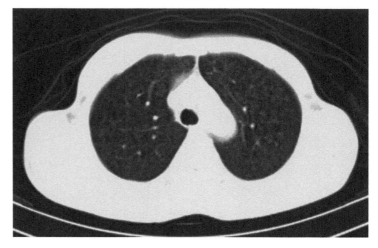

◼ **Fig. 22.1** Thoracic CT scan (Pulmonary window). Micronodular opacity focus on both lungs

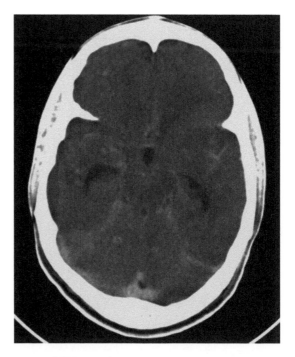

◼ **Fig. 22.2** Head CT scan with contrast

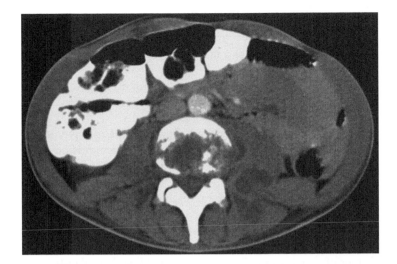

Fig. 22.3   Lumbar TC scan with contrast (soft tissue window)

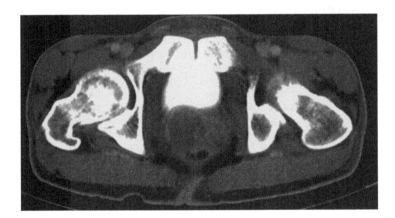

Fig. 22.4   Pelvic CT scan with contrast (soft tissue window). Prostatic abscess

Diagnosis   Pulmonary tuberculosis with extrapulmonary involvement (CNS, musculoskeletal and genitourinary)

✔ Answers to the Questions

1. Micronodular opacity focus on both lungs, multiple micronodular contrast enhancement foci scattered in the brain parenchyma, expansive lesion with involvement of the intersomatic disc, erosion of adjacent vertebral platforms and compression of the thecal sac, abscess of the psoas and spinal erector muscles and prostatic abscess.

2. Patients with «typical» imaging findings of tuberculosis are usually treated empirically; however, some cases of CNS tuberculosis have an appearance which makes them difficult to distinguish from meningitis, toxoplasmosis, lymphoma and neurosarcoidosis.

22.1 Discussion

Tuberculosis (TB) remains a major global public health problem of considerable magnitude.

We describe a case of a young patient with no positive result for HIV infection, followed for months for headache and lower back pain, with no significant improvement.

The imaging evaluation suggested the hypothesis of pulmonary and extrapulmonary TB. Following surgical decompression of the paravertebral abscess (with subsequent histopathology), antituberculosis therapy was initiated.

The patient improved and was discharged.

The present case highlights the role of imaging in the diagnosis of a disease which, though common in our environment, still poses many challenges for diagnosis, particularly with regard to the limitations of imaging as well as laboratory and histological tests.

References

1. Burrill J, Williams CJ, Bain G, et al. Tuberculosis. A radiologic review. RSNA. 2007;25(5):1255–74. Available on: http://pubs.rsna.org.
2. Rock RB, Olin M, Baker CA, et al. Central nervous system tuberculosis: pathogenesis and clinical aspects. Clin Microbiol Rev. 2008;21(2):243–61. Available on: http://cmr.asm.org.
3. Nelson CA, Zunt JR. Tuberculosis of the central nervous system in the immunocompromised patients: HIV infection and solid organ transplant recipients. CID. 2011;53(9):915–26. Available on: http://cid.oxfordjournals.org.
4. Capone D, Mogami R, Lopes AJ, et al. Extrapulmonary tuberculosis, Magazine of Pedro Ernesto University Hospital, UERJ. 2006;5(2). Available on: http://revista.hupe.uerj.br.

Brain Tumours

Contents

Case 23

Ângelo Carneiro

© Springer International Publishing AG 2018
J. Xavier et al. (eds.), *Diagnostic and Therapeutic Neuroradiology*,
https://doi.org/10.1007/978-3-319-61140-2_23

23

A 55-year-old woman presented with multiple right-hemisphere transient ischemic attacks. She had a known right cavernous sinus lesion.

❓ Questions

1. What are the findings on MR?
2. If this lesion was a pituitary adenoma, what would you expect regarding the internal carotid artery (ICA) diameter?
3. Which ICA branches are nourishing this lesion?

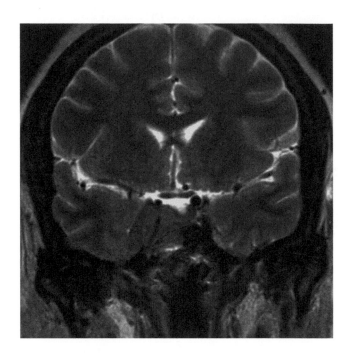

◘ **Fig. 23.1**   Coronal T2WI

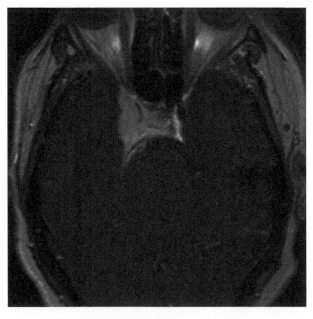

◘ **Fig. 23.2**   Axial contrast-enhanced T1WI

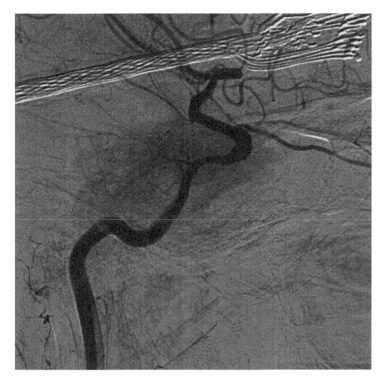

Fig. 23.3   DSA; right ICA injection, lateral view

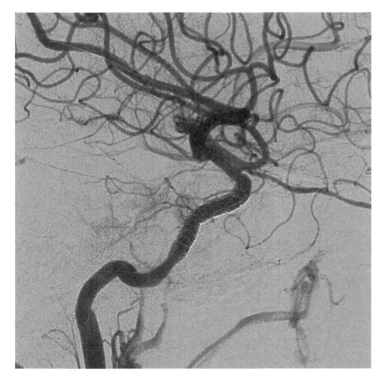

Fig. 23.4   Right ICA injection, after treatment

23

Diagnosis   Cavernous sinus meningioma with symptomatic ICA stenosis

✓ Answers to Questions

1. There is a mass in the right cavernous sinus, partially extending into the sella turcica but apparently separated/individualized from the pituitary gland (■ Fig. 23.1). It exhibits intense and homogeneous contrast enhancement and a «dural tail» (■ Fig. 23.2). The lesion encases the ICA and causes an important narrowing (compare the diameter of right versus left ICA on T2WI).
2. Pituitary adenomas can sometimes invade the cavernous sinus, surrounding the ICA. However, due to their softer consistency, they seldom cause carotid stenosis.
3. The meningioma receives arterial supply from the meningo-hypophyseal trunk (MHT) and from the inferolateral trunk (ILT) of the cavernous segment of the ICA; in this case there were no nourishing branches arising from the external carotid artery (viz., from the internal maxillary artery). Meningiomas tend to exhibit a characteristic early and intense blush on angiographic studies (■ Fig. 23.3) which usually persists; this has been called the *mother-in-law* sign («comes early, stays late»).

23.1   Comments and Discussion

Cavernous sinus meningiomas may be totally asymptomatic. Symptoms are usually related to the neurovascular structures involved. Patients most frequently present with ocular symptoms, such as diplopia, ophthalmoplegia, ptosis or anisocoria due to compression of the III, IV or VI nerves. Whenever tumours extend into the suprasellar cistern and compress the optic nerve and/or chiasm, visual field deficits or decreased visual acuity may occur. Facial numbness or pain may also ensue due to V nerve involvement [1].

Cavernous sinus meningiomas frequently cause ICA encasement and narrowing (reported incidence between 8 and 100%); however, hypoperfusion symptoms related to the stenosis are rare [2].

This patient had been submitted to radiosurgery 7 years earlier but the tumour continued to enlarge. ICA stenosis had been noticed in previous follow-up examinations but at that time it was asymptomatic. By the time it became symptomatic (with TIAs), a multidisciplinary discussion was undertaken with a decision to address the arterial stenosis. Pretreatment angiography showed 60% stenosis of the ICA (■ Fig. 23.3), with partial compensation through the circle of Willis. The patient was medicated with dual antiplatelet therapy, and, after 5 days, a balloon-mounted stent (Channel® 3.5 × 20 mm) was deployed across the stenosis. Immediate control angiogram showed a fair reconstitution of the arterial diameter, with the stent fully opened (■ Fig. 23.4). After 6 months, clopidogrel was stopped but aspirin was continued for life. Two-year follow-up (not shown) revealed no recurrent stenosis and no further TIAs occurred.

References

1. Rees J. Meningeal neoplasms. In: Naidich T, et al., editors. Imaging of the brain. Philadelphia: Elsevier Saunders; 2013. p. 642–78.
2. Heye S, et al. Symptomatic stenosis of the cavernous portion of the internal carotid artery due to an irresectable medial sphenoid wing meningioma: treatment by endovascular stent placement. Am J Neuroradiol. 2006;27(7):1532–4.

Case 24

Mariana C. Diogo, Joana T. Pinto, and Carla Conceição

© Springer International Publishing AG 2018
J. Xavier et al. (eds.), *Diagnostic and Therapeutic Neuroradiology*,
https://doi.org/10.1007/978-3-319-61140-2_24

A pregnant woman was referred for foetal MRI at 32 gestational weeks (GW) after a temporal mass was detected on ultrasound and a haemorrhage was suspected. The pregnancy had been followed appropriately, and there was no relevant personal or family history. The parents decided to carry the pregnancy to term, and the infant was re-imaged in the neonatal period.

❓ Questions

1. What are the differential diagnoses?
2. What are the main diagnostic clues?
3. What is the degree of malignancy?

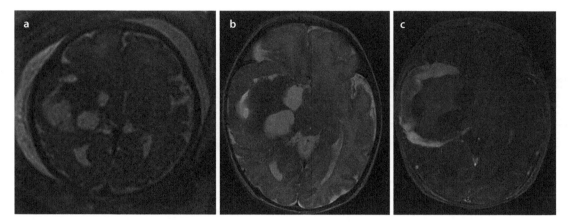

☐ **Fig. 24.1** **a** Foetal MRI at 32GW. Axial T2WI depicts a heterogeneous mass of the temporal lobe, with hypo- and hyperintense components. **b** Postnatal MRI. T2 WI. Intra-axial space-occupying lesion of the temporal lobe, heterogeneous, with solid and cystic components. There is no significant perilesional oedema and there is thinning of the adjacent skull vault. **c** Postcontrast T1 WI shows heterogeneous enhancement, mainly peripheral, with discrete adjacent dural enhancement

Diagnosis Desmoplastic infantile ganglioglioma

✅ **Answers to the Questions**

1. Differential diagnoses: pleomorphic xanthoastrocytoma, atypical teratoid/rhabdoid tumour (AT/RT), primitive neuroectodermal tumour (PNET), supratentorial ependymoma, solid and pilocytic astrocytoma.
2. Diagnostic clues: exuberant cystic components, age, absence of calcifications and preferential peripheral enhancement, extending to dura.
3. Low grade (WHO grade I).

24.1 Comments

Desmoplastic infantile ganglioglioma (DIG) is a low-grade (WHO grade I) intracranial neoplasm, occurring in infants under 2 years of age. Unlike most brain tumours in this age group, they have a typically benign course. They are large, partially cystic tumours, involving superficial cerebral cortex with invasion of the leptomeninges, and are more frequently frontal or parietal. The solid component is typically T2 hypointense, and there is an enhancement of adjacent meninges. Calcification and hemorrhagic foci are usually absent [1].

Clinically, DIG presents with increasing head circumference, bulging of the fontanels and non-specific symptoms such as seizures and vomiting, of short duration, suggesting a rather rapid growth rate of the underlying intracranial tumour.

Total resection is the treatment of choice, without the need for further adjuvant therapy.

Reference

1. Alexiou GA, Stefanaki K, Sfakianos G, Prodromou N. Desmoplastic infantile ganglioglioma. Pediatr Neurosurg. 2008;44:422–5.

Case 25

Marta Rodrigues, Antónia Furtado, and Joana Nunes

© Springer International Publishing AG 2018
J. Xavier et al. (eds.), *Diagnostic and Therapeutic Neuroradiology*,
https://doi.org/10.1007/978-3-319-61140-2_25

25

A 40-year-old woman, with no relevant clinical background, went to the emergency service with headache, nausea, vomiting and behavioural changes, without fever. Neurological examination was normal. The computed tomography (CT) revealed an expansive lesion with ventricular involvement (◘ Fig. 25.1).

? Questions
1. What are the imaging findings?
2. What are the possible differential diagnoses?
3. Which other relevant results of additional investigation are present?

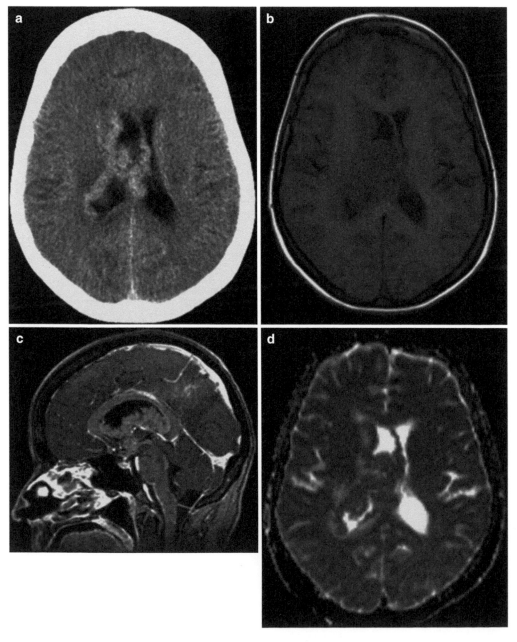

◘ **Fig. 25.1**   **a** Non-enhanced CT. **b** Axial T1. **c** Sagittal T1 Gad+. **d** Axial ADC map

Diagnosis Primary central nervous system (CNS) amelanotic melanoma

✓ Answers to Questions

1. Expansive-infiltrative lesion centred on the ependyma of the right lateral ventricle and septum pellucidum, with extension to the third and fourth ventricles and with diffuse leptomeningeal dissemination, including the facial-acoustic bundle. It is spontaneously hyperdense on CT, with post-contrast enhancement and restricted diffusion.
2. Ependymoma; lymphoproliferative disease; astrocytic tumour; central neurocytoma; choroid plexus tumour; metastatic disease; granulomatous/infectious disease.
3. Hematologic workup and cerebrospinal fluid (CSF) analysis (normal results were obtained), imaging of other organs (no evidence of other organ involvement) and anatomic-pathology study (findings consistent with melanoma lesion).

25.1 Comments

Primary malignant melanoma of the CNS accounts for approximately 1% of all melanoma cases, being most frequent in adults with a mean age of 50 years [1, 2]. This diagnosis can only be made after exclusion of secondary metastatic disease from a cutaneous, mucosal or retinal origin. Amelanotic melanoma of CNS is an extremely rare subtype [2]. It most often arises within the leptomeninges, but development within the ventricles has been reported. In the described case, the restricted diffusion on MR, the densitometric characteristics on CT and the leptomeningeal dissemination suggested lymphoproliferative disease or high-grade astrocytic tumour. The extension to the ventricular system could also indicate ependymoma. Central neurocytoma is characteristically non-infiltrative, with well-defined limits and benign morphology. Melanoma was not considered as a probable initial hypothesis due to the lack of characteristic high signal of melanin on T1-weighted images. Clinical examination and workup study (including CSF) were not consistent with granulomatous, infectious or metastatic disease. With confirmation of the pathologic study, and since no other melanoma lesion was evident on physical examination, diagnosis of primary CNS melanoma was made.

References

1. Wadasadawala T, Trivedi S, Gupta T, Epari S, Jalali R. The diagnostic dilemma of primary central nervous system melanoma. J Clin Neurosci. 2010;17:1014–7.
2. Ma J, Zhang Z, Li S, Chen X, Wang S. Intracranial amelanotic melanoma: a case report with literature review. World J Surg Oncol. 2015;13:182.

Case 26

Vasco Pinto, Mário Gomes, Manuel Melo Pires, and Carla Silva

© Springer International Publishing AG 2018
J. Xavier et al. (eds.), *Diagnostic and Therapeutic Neuroradiology*,
https://doi.org/10.1007/978-3-319-61140-2_26

A 52-year-old woman presents with gradually progressive head-aches and discrete motor dysphasia, with 6 months of evolution.

? Questions

1. What are the findings on these MRI images?
2. What are the relevant differential diagnoses?
3. What other imaging studies would be useful for further treatment planning?

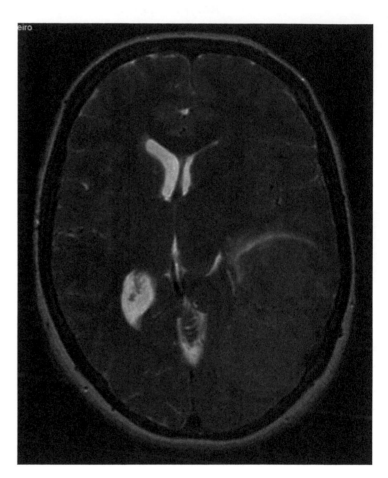

◘ Fig. 26.1   Axial T2 fast-recovery fast spin echo

Case 26

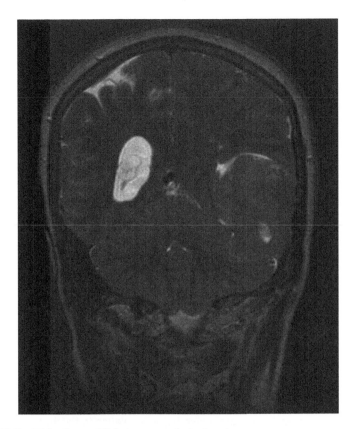

Fig. 26.2   Coronal T2 fast-recovery fast spin echo

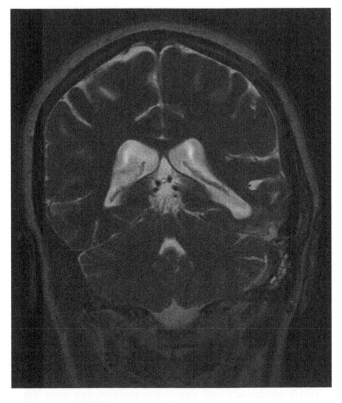

Fig. 26.3   Coronal T2 fast-recovery fast spin echo, post-op

26

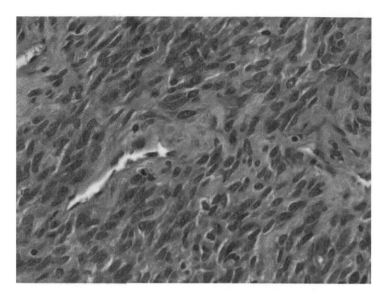

◧ **Fig. 26.4**   H&E of the lesion, 40× amplification, optical microscopy

Diagnosis   Primary intracranial solitary fibrous tumour/hemangiopericytoma

✅ **Answers to Questions**
1. In ◧ Figs. 26.1 and 26.2, an extra-axial, lobulated, temporo-occipital space-occupying lesion in relation to the tentorium cerebelli, with a probable infratentorial component may be observed. It measures 79.4 × 57.5 × 55.1 mm and locally collapses the lateral ventricle and causes a 5 mm midline shift. It presents slight signal heterogeneity, with an isointense to discreetly hyperintense background with small hypointense areas. ◧ Figure 26.3 is a postsurgical exeresis image, with a left temporal T2 hyperintense area, cortex loss and left ventricular ex vacuo dilatation. In ◧ Fig. 26.4, a neoplasm can be identified, with evidence of hyperchromatic nests, some pleomorphism and a spindle-cellular pattern. A few mitoses are present.
2. Meningioma; solitary fibrous tumour.
3. TOF MR angiography for evaluation of anatomical relations with and patency of dural venous sinuses for surgical planning, as an example.

26.1   Comments

Primary CNS solitary fibrous tumours (now more properly denominated solitary fibrous tumours/hemangiopericytomas (SFT/HPCs) according to the new 2016 WHO CNS tumours classification) are rare mesenchymal neoplasms, accounting for approximately 0.09% of meningeal tumours [1]. Diagnosis is centrally dependent on histology, as clinical and imaging evaluation lacks specificity [1, 2]. SFT/HPCs are usually well-defined masses arising from the dura.

Over half exhibit isointense signal on T1W imaging, over half exhibit a T2W hypointense signal and over three quarters enhance with gadolinium. The differential is complex, with SFT/HPCs often misdiagnosed (even after histology) as meningioma, fibrous histiocytoma and fibrosarcoma [1]. Treatment rests on surgical resection and the prognosis is good with gross total removal. There is little evidence supporting adjuvant chemotherapy or radiotherapy [1, 2].

References

1. Wang Z, et al. Intracranial solitary fibrous tumors: a report of two cases and a review of the literature. Oncol Lett. 2016;11(2):1057–60.
2. Metellus P, et al. Solitary fibrous tumors of the CNS: clinicopathological and therapeutic considerations of 18 cases. Neurosurgery. 2007;60(4):715–22.

Case 27

Luís Cardoso, Luís Albuquerque, and Cristina Ramos

© Springer International Publishing AG 2018
J. Xavier et al. (eds.), *Diagnostic and Therapeutic Neuroradiology*,
https://doi.org/10.1007/978-3-319-61140-2_27

A 59-year-old male, with recent diagnosis of high-grade glioma in the right motor area. The patient underwent surgery with subtotal removal of the lesion followed by chemoradiotherapy. Images below represent MR imaging before surgery (◘ Figs. 27.1 and 27.2) and after completion of chemoradiotherapy protocol (◘ Figs. 27.3 and 27.4).

❓ Questions

1. Describe the MR findings.
2. Why is it important to maintain surveillance over these patients?
3. Are there other MR techniques which might be useful for the evaluation?

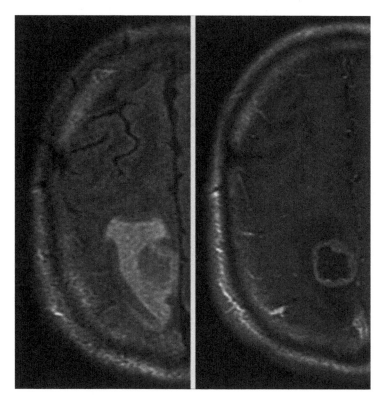

◘ **Fig. 27.1**   Axial FLAIR/T1 + contrast – initial

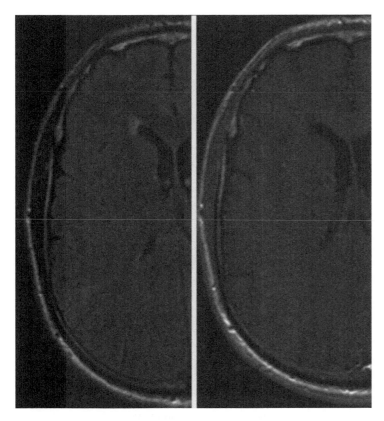

◘ **Fig. 27.2** Axial FLAIR/T1 + contrast – initial

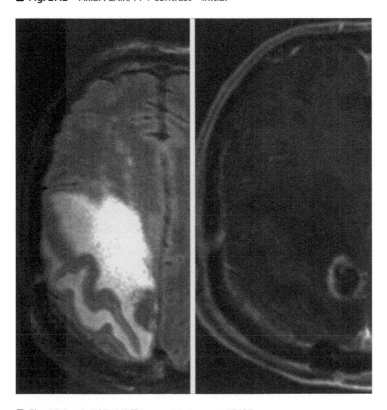

◘ **Fig. 27.3** Axial FLAIR/T1 + contrast – post RT/QT

27

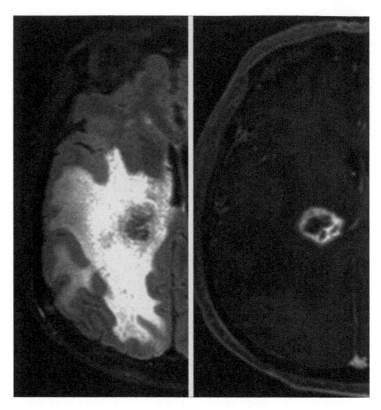

Fig. 27.4   Axial FLAIR/T1 + contrast – post RT/QT

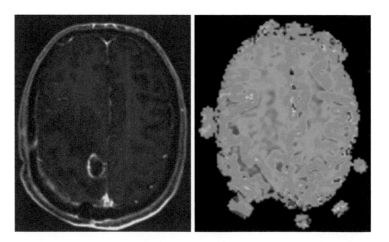

Fig. 27.5   Axial T1 + contrast and rCBV map – post RT/QT; high perfusion on rCBV map on the corresponding enhancing lesion

Diagnosis   Glioblastoma - Tumour Recurrence

✅ **Answers to Questions**

1. A right frontoparietal parasagittal ring-enhancing lesion surrounded by hyperintense vasogenic oedema on FLAIR, with central necrosis on contrast T1-weighted image (◼ Fig. 27.1). Post-treatment imaging shows a larger lesion in the same previously enhancing area (◼ Fig. 27.3) and, additionally, a de novo right periventricular enhancing lesion, with central necrosis and increased perfusion on rCBV maps, suggesting tumour progression (◼ Figs. 27.4 and 27.5). There is an overall enlargement of the hyperintense nonenhancing white matter changes on FLAIR, likely due to coexisting oedema, post-radiation leukoencephalopathy and tumoural infiltration.

2. Recurrent tumours and treatment-related changes frequently have overlapping clinical and radiological features. Both may evolve with new or increasing enhancing mass lesions and may follow criteria for progression. This differentiation can be difficult and requires follow-up imaging, with the changes related to pseudoprogression becoming stable or decreasing in size.

3. DSC-MR perfusion, DWI and spectroscopy may be useful in differentiating recurrent tumour from treatment-related changes or pseudoprogression, but further studies are required.

27.1 Comments

Contrast enhancement after brain tumour treatment is nonspecific and may not always be considered an adequate assessment for tumour response or recurrence [1]. Pseudoprogression (an increase in the nontumoural enhancing area) and pseudoresponse (a decrease in the enhancing area) suggest that enhancement, by itself, is mostly a consequence of a disturbed blood-brain barrier, confusing outcome evaluation and sometimes causing erroneous changes in therapy. Histopathological studies show that treatment-related changes are characterised by vascular dilation, endothelial damage and fibrinoid necrosis of normal vasculature, whereas a recurrent tumour is marked by the presence of increased cellularity, tumour cells and vascular proliferation [1, 2]. Distinction may be achieved by follow-up examinations, with pseudoprogression occurring predominantly within the first 12 weeks after completing treatment, though it can also endure up to 6 months after treatment. Perfusion MR imaging is an additional technique which provides information on neoangiogenesis, microvascular leakiness and vascular attenuation. Cases of recurrent tumours confirmed after repeated surgery were associated with hyperperfusion on rCBV map, while treatment-related changes were described as having higher DWI and lower perfusion on rCBV map [1].

References

1. Prager AJ, Martinez N, Beal K, Omuro A, Zhang Z, Young RJ. Diffusion and perfusion MRI to differentiate treatment- related changes including pseudoprogression from recurrent tumors in high-grade gliomas with histopathologic evidence. AJNR Neuroradiology. 2015;36(5):877–85.
2. Hygino da Cruz LC, Rodriguez I, Domingues RC, Gasparetto EL, Sorensen AG. Pseudoprogression and pseudoresponse: imaging challenges in the assessment of posttreatment glioma. AJNR. 2011;32(11):1978–85.

27

Case 28

Nuno Ferreira Silva

© Springer International Publishing AG 2018
J. Xavier et al. (eds.), *Diagnostic and Therapeutic Neuroradiology*,
https://doi.org/10.1007/978-3-319-61140-2_28

A 60-year-old woman, in follow-up of a left frontal glioblastoma, diagnosed in the setting of a first seizure, with subsequent MRI investigation, maximal safe surgical resection and first-line treatment with radiotherapy and concurrent and adjuvant temozolomide (Stupp protocol). Below, pre-surgical (◘ Figs. 28.1 and 28.2), first 48-h period after surgery (◘ Fig. 28.3), 3 months post-radiotherapy (◘ Figs. 28.4 and 28.5), and 22 months post-radiotherapy (◘ Fig. 28.6) studies.

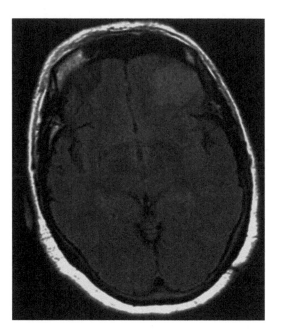

◘ Fig. 28.1   Axial T2 FLAIR

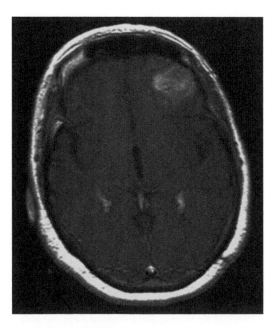

◘ Fig. 28.2   Post-enhanced T1WI

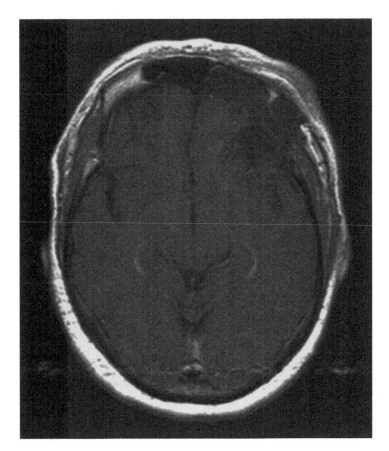

◘ **Fig. 28.3**   Post-enhanced T1WI

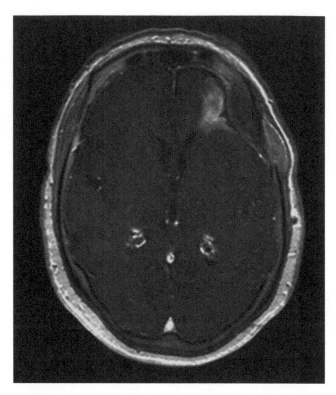

Fig. 28.4   Post-enhanced T1WI

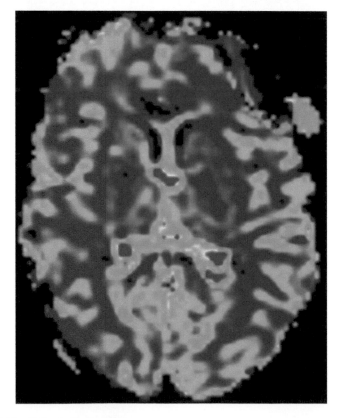

Fig. 28.5   Perfusion (CBV)

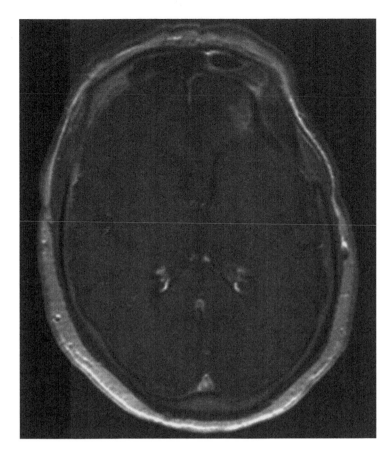

■ **Fig. 28.6**   Post-enhanced T1WI

❓ Questions

1. What is the purpose of an early baseline MRI scan after surgery?
2. What could ■ Fig. 28.4 stand for, and relying on perfusion study (■ Fig. 28.5), which possibility would better explain it?
3. Does ■ Fig. 28.6 support perfusion study and hence what is the diagnosis?

Diagnosis   Glioblastoma pseudoprogression

✅ Answers

1. Increased enhancement in the margins of the surgical cavity, not related to the tumour itself (postoperative changes), frequently takes place 48–72 h after resection. Thus, to avoid misinterpreted residual enhancement disease, baseline MRI is recommended within 24–48 h after surgery.
2. At this point, contrast enhancement could relate to tumour progression or post-radiation changes, the latter being more plausible, as no increase in perfusion was found (exactly the opposite of previous case – ▶ Chap. 27).
3. Reduction in contrast enhancement is consistent with post-radiation changes, as the perfusion study suggested.

28.1 Comments

Twenty to thirty percent of patients under Stupp protocol reveal transient contrast enhancement after radiotherapy completion [1], likely due to secondary increased tumour vasculature permeability (which may be reinforced by temozolomide) [1, 2, 3]. This effect, known as pseudoprogression and sometimes accompanied by clinical decline, is more frequent within the first 12 weeks [1, 2, 3], eventually subsiding with no additional measures. Given the implications in patients' management, short-term clinical and MRI follow-up is required, also taking into account T2/FLAIR signal abnormality response, as well as additional data provided by diffusion, perfusion and spectroscopy.

References

1. Wen PY, et al. Updated response assessment criteria for high-grade gliomas: response assessment in neuro-oncology working group. J Clin Oncol. 2010;28(11):1963–72.
2. da Cruz LCH, et al. Pseudoprogression and pseudoresponse: imaging challenges in the assessment of posttreatment glioma. Am J Neuroradiol. 2011;32(11):1978–85.
3. Linhares P, et al. Early pseudoprogression following chemoradiotherapy in glioblastoma patients: the value of RANO evaluation. J Oncol. 2013;2013:1–9.

28

Case 29

Eleonora Kvasceviciene and Robertas Kvascevicius

© Springer International Publishing AG 2018
J. Xavier et al. (eds.), *Diagnostic and Therapeutic Neuroradiology*,
https://doi.org/10.1007/978-3-319-61140-2_29

A 63-year-old white woman had a flu episode, from which she recovered with some complaints but several months later developed severe headaches, weakness, shimmering and blurred vision, language apprehension difficulties, slight weakness and numbness in the left arm and leg.

? Questions

1. What are the findings?
2. What are the differential diagnoses in this case?
3. What kind of action is suggested in this case?

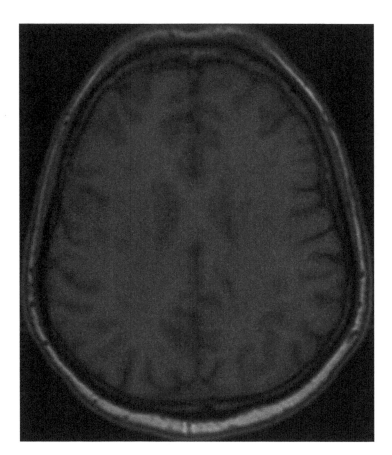

◘ **Fig. 29.1**   MRT axial non-enhanced T1

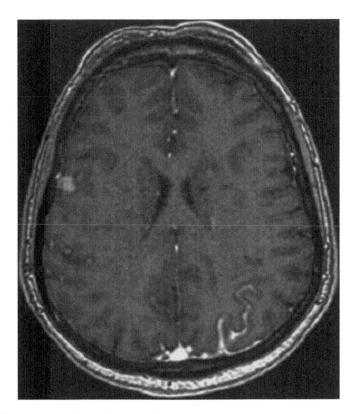

Fig. 29.2   MRT axial enhanced T1

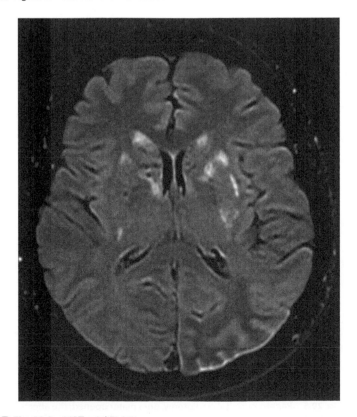

Fig. 29.3   MRT axial FLAIR

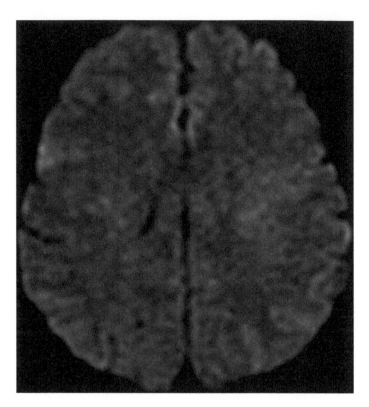

◩ **Fig. 29.4**   MRT axial DWI

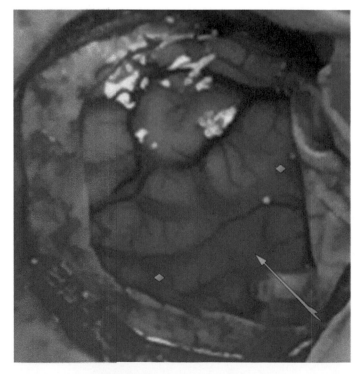

◩ **Fig. 29.5**   Parieto-occipital craniotomy, dura mater opened, the affected parietal gyri are visible through the arachnoidal layer (*blue arrow* and *dots*)

Diagnosis Primary CNS lymphoplasmacytic lymphoma (non-Hodgkin lymphoma)

✔ **Answers**

1. ◻ Figure 29.1 – MRT axial non-enhanced T1: filling of the left occipital sulci with isointense content, isointense dural-based mass in the right frontal region.

    ◻ Figure 29.2 – MRT axial enhanced T1: prominent leptomeningeal enhancement in the sulci of the left occipital lobe, enhanced dural-based mass in the right frontal region.

    ◻ Figure 29.3 – MRT axial FLAIR: hyperintensities in the sulci and meninges of the left occipital lobe, diffuse hypointensities in the subcortical white matter of the left occipital lobe, multiple hyperintense foci along prominent Robin-Virchow space in the basal ganglia.

    ◻ Figure 29.4 – MRT axial DWI: restricted diffusion in the dural-based mass in the right frontal lobe.

2. Secondary CNS lymphoma, meningeal carcinomatosis, neurosarcoidosis, infectious/granulomatous meningitis and leptomeningeal melanosis.

3. After clinical and general investigation, one of the CNS lymphomas was suspected and the patient was investigated in the haematological service, where bone marrow biopsy and body PET/CT revealed no systemic lymphoma. Open brain biopsy was performed (craniotomy and partial resection of affected gyrus with leptomeninges and cortical-subcortical small vessels). Histology: Non-Hodgkin lymphoma, B lymphoplasmacytic lymphoma (immunophenotypic profile CD20+, BCL2+, CD138+, CD38+, IgM and IgG positive membrane reaction, Ki-67 –5%; negative immunohist. reactions: CD5, CD3 CD23, BCL6, CD10, cyclin D1, IgD; AmyAA; FISH: MYD88 mutation negative) (◻ Fig. 29.5).

29.1 Comments

Lymphoplasmacytic lymphoma is a chronic lymphoproliferative disorder characterized by a proliferation of plasma cells, small lymphocytes, plasmacytoid lymphocytes and the production of monoclonal IgM. Primary central nervous system lymphomas (PCNSL) are rare non-Hodgkin lymphomas (NHL), accounting for only 2–3% of NHL cases [1]. The diffuse form corresponds to lymphoid cell infiltration in the leptomeningeal sheaths and the perivascular spaces, and usually presents with contrast enhancement and/or thickening of meningeal sheaths [2]. Although MRI is a very sensitive technique for the detection of malignant infiltration of CNS, it cannot different histological entities of CNS lymphoma [2]. Definitive diagnosis of primary CNS lymphoma requires histologic assessment [3], direct biopsy of the affected tissue is mandatory in planning appropriate treatment.

References

1. Abbi KK, Muzaffar M, Gaudin D, Booth RL Jr, Feldmeier JJ, Skeel RT, Primary CNS. lymphoplasmacytic lymphoma:a case report and review of literature. Hematol oncol Stem Cell Ther. 2013;6(2):76–8.
2. Minnema MC, et al. Guideline for the diagnosis, treatment and response criteria for Bing-Neel syndrome. Haematologica. 2017;102(1):43–51.
3. Slone HW, Blake JJ, Shah R, et al. CT and MRI findings of intracranial lymphoma. AJR Am J Roentgenol. 2005;184(5):1679–85.

29

Vascular

Contents

Case 30

Viriato Alves

© Springer International Publishing AG 2018
J. Xavier et al. (eds.), *Diagnostic and Therapeutic Neuroradiology*,
https://doi.org/10.1007/978-3-319-61140-2_30

A 27-year-old woman woke up with right hemiparesis and dysphasia (NIHSS 13). Normal CT scan.

? Questions

1. What are the findings on these images?
2. What are the possible aetiologies?
3. Why is the treatment urgent?

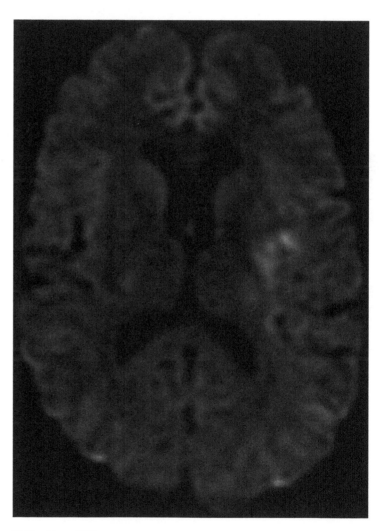

◘ **Fig. 30.1**   DWI

Case 30

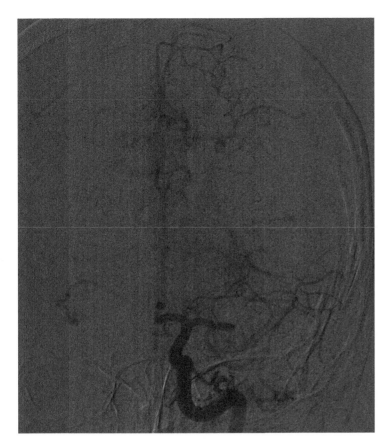

◘ **Fig. 30.2**   DSA

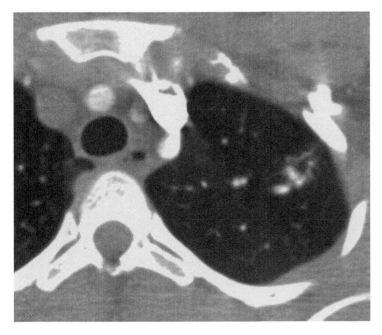

◘ **Fig. 30.3**   CT

Diagnosis   Acute ischaemic stroke in patient with hereditary haemorrhagic telangiectasia (HHT) and a pulmonary AVM

✓ Answers

1. MR ▣ Fig. 30.1 – left posterior lenticular restricted diffusion; DSA ▣ Fig. 30.2 – MCA occlusion by thrombus with collateral circulation via pial anastomoses from the ACA and anterior temporal branch of the MCA, two small bilateral temporal AVMs; thoracic CT ▣ Fig. 30.3 – pulmonary arteriovenous malformation.
2. Carotid dissection; carotid bulb atherosclerotic plaque (unlikely at this age); cardiac origin of the thrombus (patent foramen ovale, etc.).
3. Mechanical thrombectomy performed in an early phase will allow reperfusion of the ischaemic penumbra territory, reverting the neurological deficits; if the patient is treated in a late phase, the recanalisation will be futile, with no improvement of the neurological deficits and with an added risk of haemorrhagic transformation of the infarct.

Post-thrombectomy Images (▣ Figs. 30.4 and 30.5)

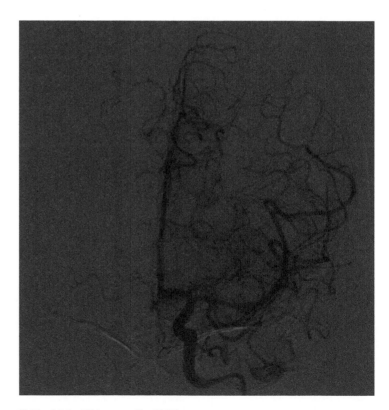

▣ **Fig. 30.4**   DSA, recanalised MCA

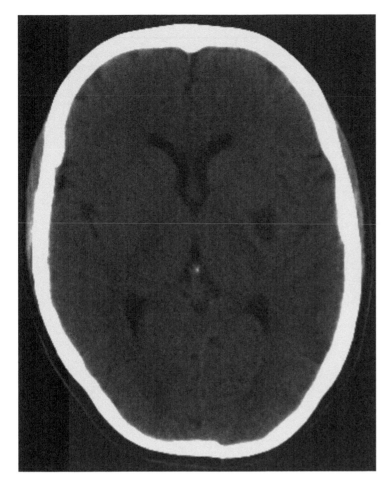

◻ Fig. 30.5   CT, posterior lenticular infarct

30.1 Comments

Hereditary haemorrhagic telangiectasia, also known as HHT or Osler-Weber-Rendu syndrome, is an autosomal dominant disorder with mucocutaneous telangiectasias and AVMs in visceral organs (primarily lungs, brain and liver) [1]. The most common clinical presentation is recurrent epistaxis from nasal mucosal telangiectasias. There is a significant lifetime risk of a brain abscess or stroke if a pulmonary AVM is present, as occurred with this patient. Pulmonary AVMs can be treated by embolisation or surgery with excellent results [2]. Most cerebral AVMs in HHT are low grade (Spetzler-Martin 1 or 2) and have a lower bleeding risk than sporadic AVMs. They can be treated with embolisation or radiosurgery, depending on the size and location of the AVM.

References

1. Krings T, et al. Neurovascular manifestations in hereditary hemorrhagic telangiectasia: imaging features and genotype-phenotype correlations. AJNR Am J Neuroradiol. 2015;36(5):863–70.
2. Osborn AG, Salzman KL, Jhaveri MD. Diagnostic imaging: brain. 3rd ed. Philadelphia: Elsiever; 2016.

Case 31

Luís Albuquerque and José Pedro Rocha Pereira

© Springer International Publishing AG 2018
J. Xavier et al. (eds.), *Diagnostic and Therapeutic Neuroradiology*,
https://doi.org/10.1007/978-3-319-61140-2_31

31.1   Clinical Information

An 80-year-old man was admitted with acute onset (3 h) of global aphasia, right homonymous hemianopsia and right hemiplegia, scoring 22 points in the NIH stroke scale.

❓ Questions
1. What are the findings?
2. How can we estimate the size of the infarct's core and the ischaemic penumbra?
3. What is the pathological mechanism behind the stroke?

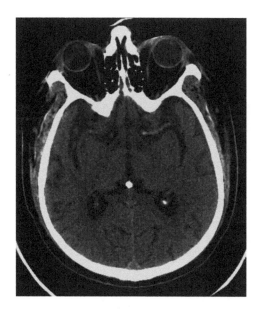

◘ Fig. 31.1   Non-contrast head CT, axial view

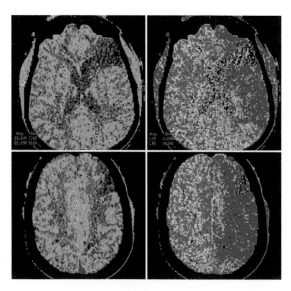

◘ Fig. 31.2   Brain perfusion CT, with CBV maps on the left and MTT maps on the right

Case 31

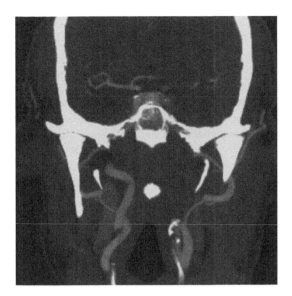

Fig. 31.3 CT angiography, coronal view of cervical and intracranial arteries

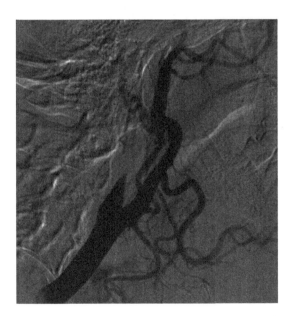

Fig. 31.4 Digital subtraction angiography, lateral view of the left carotid bifurcation

Diagnosis   Tandem acute ischaemic stroke of the left internal carotid artery (ICA) territory

✅ **Answers**

1. Non-contrast CT shows a spontaneous hyperdensity in the M1 segment of the left middle cerebral artery (MCA) (◘ Fig. 31.1) that, in this clinical context, reflects the presence of an intraluminal thrombus. Perfusion CT shows a relatively small area of reduced CBV, in the left fronto-opercular

region, and an extensive area of prolonged mean transit time (MTT), comprising the full territories of both left MCA and anterior cerebral artery (ACA) (◘ Fig. 31.2). A T-shaped thrombus is apparent in the CT angiography, extending from the terminal segment of the left ICA to the M1 and A1 segments of the respective cerebral arteries (◘ Fig. 31.3). Digital subtraction angiography shows a beak-shaped addition image immediately after the origin of the left ICA, consistent with arterial dissection (◘ Fig. 31.4).

2. CBV maps show reduced CBV on the ischaemic core. The difference between the areas with changed values in the MTT and the CBV maps gives us the ischaemic penumbra, which is potentially salvageable.

3. The initial mechanism was the left ICA dissection, which in turn formed a thrombus that embolized distally to the M1 segment of the MCA – a tandem occlusion.

31.2   After Endovascular Treatment (◘ Figs. 31.5 and 31.6)

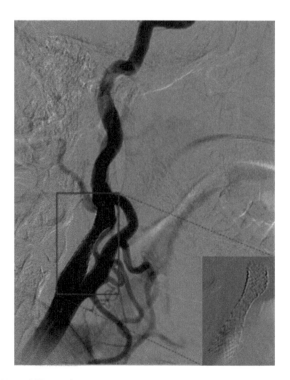

◘ Fig. 31.5   ICA stenting

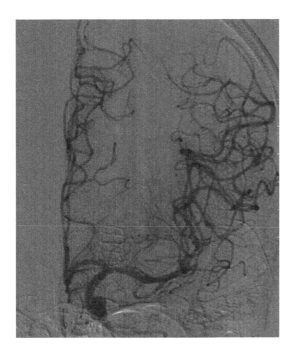

◘ Fig. 31.6 Outcome after stent-retriever thrombectomy

31.3 Comments

Presently, mechanical thrombectomy along with IV thrombolysis is the standard recommended treatment for patients presenting with ischaemic stroke and a large-vessel occlusion [1]. Numerous trials have proved the benefit of this technique. Cervical internal carotid artery occlusion (either atherosclerotic or by dissection) can pose a technical challenge for this approach, as it decreases the efficacy of the IV tPA [2] and represents an obstacle to catheter navigation, but it is not a contra-indication for this technique.

In this case, the patient was first treated with IV tPA, with no significant clinical changes. In the angiography room, the left ICA dissection was successfully navigated through, followed by removal of the thrombus lodged at the top of the artery with a stent retriever (◘ Fig. 31.6). Afterwards, the ICA dissection was approached, with placement of a metallic stent in order to maintain the vessel's patency (◘ Fig. 31.5). The patient had a favourable outcome and was asymptomatic at the time of medical discharge, despite having a fronto-opercular infarct.

References

1. Powers J, et al. AHA/ASA focused update of the 2013 guidelines for the early management of patients with Acute Ischemic Stroke regarding endovascular treatment. Stroke. 2015;46:3020–35.
2. Lavallée PC, et al. Stent-assisted endovascular thrombolysis vs. intravenous thrombolysis in internal carotid artery dissection with tandem internal carotid and middle cerebral artery occlusion. Stroke. 2007;38:2270–4.

Case 32

Luís Albuquerque, Ângelo Carneiro, and João Xavier

© Springer International Publishing AG 2018
J. Xavier et al. (eds.), *Diagnostic and Therapeutic Neuroradiology*,
https://doi.org/10.1007/978-3-319-61140-2_32

32.1 Clinical Information

A 69-year-old male patient, with a history of multiple lumbar spine surgeries due to lumbar canal stenosis, presenting with lower back pain, paraparesis and paresthesia, associated with urinary incontinence.

? **Questions**
1. Describe the MR findings.
2. Name the arterial structures present in the left image of ◘ Fig. 32.2.
3. Is there a therapeutic indication?

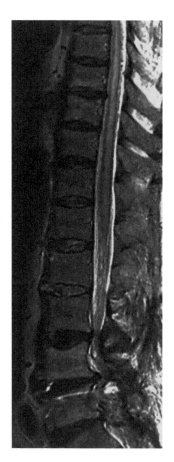

◘ **Fig. 32.1**   MR, T2 sagittal view

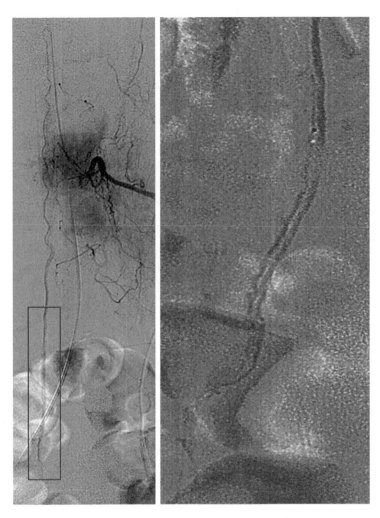

□ Fig. 32.2 *Left* Digital subtraction angiography, PA views of contrast injections in L1 segmental artery; *Right* Close-up of an injection at the same level

Diagnosis   Arteriovenous fistula of the filum terminale

✅ Answers

1. Intramedullary increased T2 signal from D7 to the conus medullaris, perimedullary flow voids and signs of previous lumbar spine surgery and disc disease (□ Fig. 32.1).
2. In order: L1 segmental artery, artery of Adamkiewicz ("hairpin"-like vessel), anterior spinal artery, artery of the filum terminale (□ Fig. 32.2 left).
3. Yes. Spinal cord venous congestion indicates treatment by exclusion of the A-V shunt, which may be accomplished by endovascular or surgical approach.

32.2   Comments

The filum terminale is a thin strand of connective fibrous tissue that extends from apex of the conus medullaris and attaches to the dorsal coccyx, providing structural support for the spinal cord [1]. It has an internal and external section – the proximal three quarters are covered by dura and arachnoid and constitute the internal section ending at the dura's cul-de-sac at S2 level [1]. Its arterial supply derives from the artery of the filum terminale, which arises from the anterior spinal artery, after passing the conus basket. The venous drainage is accomplished through the vein of the filum terminale, which connects to the extradural sacral venous plexus and to the ventral vein of the spinal cord.

Arteriovenous fistulas of the filum terminale are extremely rare with uncertain incidence. Its symptoms derive mainly from spinal cord venous congestion and may range from mild back pain to severe neurological deficits. In this patient's case, the history of lumbar surgeries could act as a confounding factor to the diagnosis. Treatment can be either endovascular or surgical, depending on the complexity of the fistula. More complex fistulae, with tortuous vessels, multiple feeders or complex venous drainage are preferably treated by surgery, while fistulae with a single feeder and a single draining vein can be successfully approached by endovascular procedure.

This patient's fistula was treated by endovascular embolisation with glue, after feeder catheterisation just proximal to the shunt (◘ Fig. 32.3 left). ◘ Figure 32.3 right shows exclusion of the fistula and patency of the anterior spinal artery. Over the following 3 weeks, there was a slight improvement of the neurological deficits and control MR revealed spinal cord oedema reduction and no perimedullary flow voids (◘ Fig. 32.4 left and right).

32.3 After Endovascular Treatment

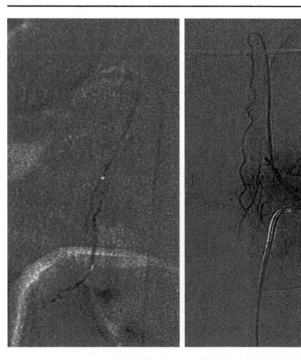

◘ **Fig. 32.3** *Left* Cast of glue after removing microcatheter (note the white spot indicating its previous position); *Right* Control injection at L1 segmental artery, showing the end result

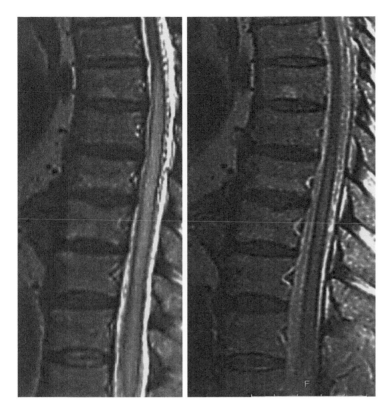

◘ **Fig. 32.4** *Left* MRI before treatment; *Right* 3 weeks after embolization: note the decrease in T2 intramedullary signal intensity, the thickness reduction of the spinal cord and absence of flow voids

Reference

1. Lim SM, et al. Spinal Arteriovenous Fistulas of the Filum Terminale. Am J Neuroradiol. 2011;32:1846–50.

Case 33

Carla Guerreiro, Joana Tavares, and Sofia Reimão

© Springer International Publishing AG 2018
J. Xavier et al. (eds.), *Diagnostic and Therapeutic Neuroradiology*,
https://doi.org/10.1007/978-3-319-61140-2_33

A 50-year-old man, who attempted suicide by hanging, presented with upper airway lesion and cervical subcutaneous emphysema. Brain CT was unremarkable. CT angiography of the neck and subsequent catheter angiography of the carotid arteries showed the following:

? Questions

1. What are the imaging findings?
2. What are the potential complications of this condition?
3. What is the preferred treatment?

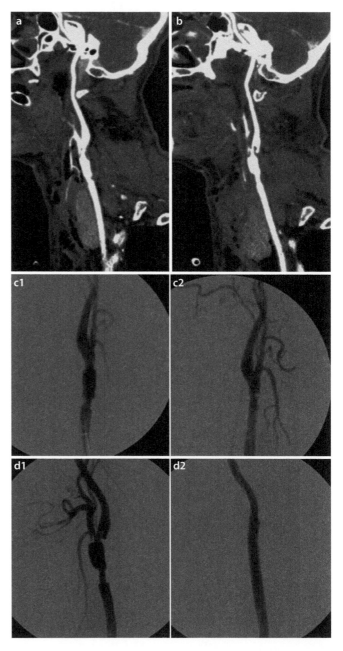

◘ Fig. 33.1 CT angiography of the neck, right **a** and left **b** parasagittal views. Subtraction angiography of right **c** and left **d** common carotid arteries, before (C1, D1) and after (C2, D2) endovascular treatment

Diagnosis   Bilateral carotid artery dissection

✅ **Answers to Questions**

1. CT angiography of the neck shows features suggestive of right (◼ Fig. 33.1a) and left (◼ Fig. 33.1b) anterior cervical arterial system dissection. «String signs» or «tie signs», translating to narrowing of the lumen, can be seen on two levels bilaterally and are reckoned to be indirect signs of artery dissection. On the right, dissection signs can be found on the common carotid artery, being the most superior point of dissection before the common carotid artery bifurcation. On the left, dissection signs are on the common carotid artery and on its bifurcation, extending horizontally from the origin of the internal carotid artery to the origin of the external carotid artery. Past the dissection points, both the internal and external carotid arteries on either side have normal morphology and patency. Catheter angiography images of the carotid arteries show right (C1, C2) and left (D1, D2) common carotids pre- (C1 and D1) and posttreatment (C2 and D2) with stenting, restoring the normal calibre of the vasa.

2. The clinical picture is usually subtle at the outset and many cases remain undetected. Complications result from primary cervical vascular injury and/or secondary ischemia [1]. Expanding intramural hematoma may present with neck and face pain, headache, and Horner syndrome, due to compression of sympathetic nerves adjacent to the internal carotid artery. Ischemic infarction/transient ischemic attacks result more commonly from distal embolization of a clot formed within the dissected vas rather than occlusion and typically occur hours to days after the onset of the dissection.

3. Asymptomatic patients with low-grade dissections are typically treated conservatively with medical management and close imaging observation [1]. However, endovascular treatment with stenting, which was the treatment of choice in this case, is becoming more popular. This minimally invasive method has shown optimal technical success, low recurrent rates, and satisfying 1-year follow-ups [1].

33.1   Discussion

Dissection and thrombotic occlusion of the carotid arteries is a rare but potentially life-threatening complication after near hanging. In hanging victims, arterial obstruction and intimal tears were found at the level of the ligature in about 5% of autopsies [2].

Dissection occurs when an intimal tear allows blood to enter the arterial wall, dividing the layers of the wall. This leads to stenosis, occlusion, or pseudoaneurysm formation.

CT angiography is frequently used for initial screening of carotid dissection, but the golden standard remains digital subtraction angiography, which permits a potential intervention via endovascular techniques when indicated [1]. However, it is an invasive method with a complication rate of almost 1%, and it is not readily available in all institutions. Both techniques have over 97% sensitivity [1].

Typical angiographic findings of dissection include luminal irregular stenosis (tie sign/ string sign), mouse's tail sign (smooth narrowing to a sharp occlusion), miointimal flaps and double lumen with an intimal flap (pathognomonic sign, which is rarely observed), and pseudoaneurysm.

References

1. Galyfos G, Filis K, Sigala F, Sianou A. Traumatic carotid artery dissection: a different entity without specific guidelines. Vasc Spec Int. 2016;32(1):1.
2. Linnau KF, Cohen WA. Radiologic evaluation of attempted suicide by hanging: cricotracheal separation and common carotid artery dissection. Am J Roentgenol 2002; 178(1):214–4.

33

Case 34

Viriato Alves

© Springer International Publishing AG 2018
J. Xavier et al. (eds.), *Diagnostic and Therapeutic Neuroradiology*,
https://doi.org/10.1007/978-3-319-61140-2_34

A 64-year-old female with sensory changes of the lower limbs, without a defined level, with about 1 year of evolution, without motor deficit, with progressive worsening and clinical deterioration in the last 6 weeks with gait disturbance and bladder incontinence.

❓ Questions
1. What are the findings on these MR and DSA images?
2. What are the differential diagnoses?
3. Why is the treatment urgent?

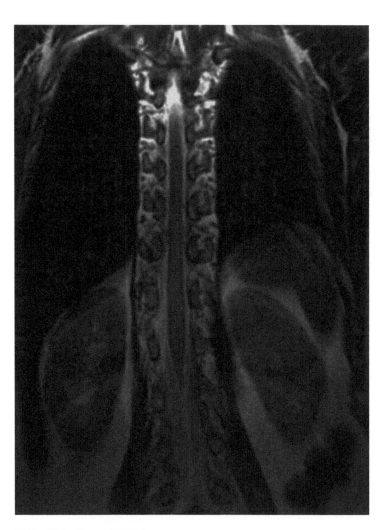

◻ **Fig. 34.1**   Coronal T2/TSE

Case 34

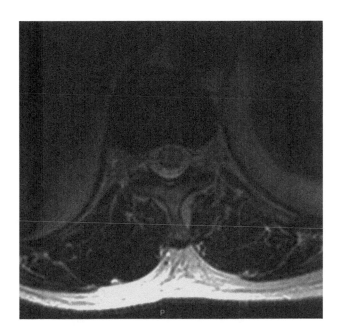

◘ Fig. 34.2   Axial T2/TSE

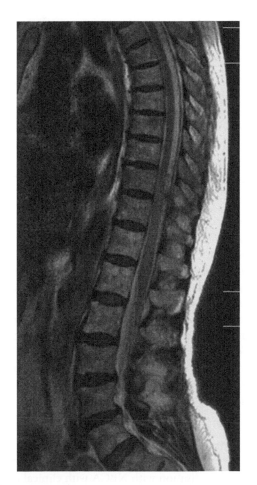

◘ Fig. 34.3   Sagittal T2/TSE

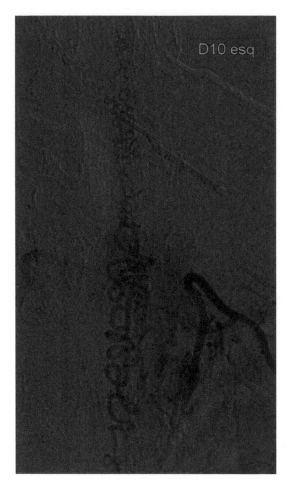

◘ Fig. 34.4 DSA

Diagnosis   Spinal arteriovenous dural fistula

✅ **Answers**
1. T2 hyperintensity of the spinal cord, sparing the periphery
    (◘ Figs. 34.1, 34.2 and 34.3); multiple intradural abnormal
    vessel flow voids (◘ Fig. 34.3). The late arterial phase DSA
    image (◘ Fig. 34.4) shows the SDAVF and the enlarged and
    tortuous spinal veins.
2. Spinal cord arteriovenous malformation (no nidus);
    collateral venous flow from inferior vena cava occlusion
    (ruled out by DSA).
3. The neurological deficits reverse if treatment is carried out
    early but become irreversible if the patient is treated in a
    late phase.

34.1   Treatment

Endovascular embolisation with NBCA with clinical improvement
(◘ Figs. 34.5 and 34.6)

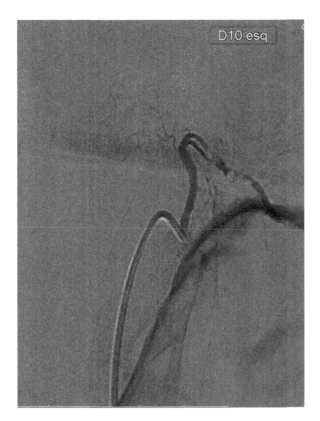

◨ **Fig. 34.5** DSA, fistula excluded

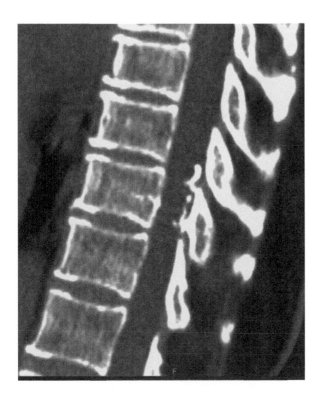

◨ **Fig. 34.6** CT, glue cast in the fistula and draining vein

34.2 **Comments**

Spinal dural arteriovenous fistulae are acquired shunts within or adjacent to the dura along the spinal canal. They cause symptoms through venous hypertension and congestion of the spinal cord with oedema. The presentation is usually in the fifth or sixth decade of life with a male predominance [1]. The most common clinical presentation is progressive paraparesis, exacerbated by exercise. Other symptoms are paresthesia, pain, bladder/bowel incontinence and impotence. Haemorrhage is rare. The time from onset of symptoms to diagnosis is often long, with the patients presenting with multiple symptoms at the medical consultation. The natural history is one of a slowly progressive clinical course, over years, ending in paraplegia. Treatment is usually performed by endovascular embolisation, occluding the fistula and proximal draining vein with a liquid embolic agent [2]. If the endovascular treatment is unsuccessful or contraindicated (patients in whom the anterior or posterior spinal arteries originate from the same level as the SDAVF), surgery should be performed during the same hospital stay.

References

1. Morris JM. Imaging of dural arteriovenous fistula. Radiol Clin N Am. 2012;50:823–39.
2. Lasjaunias P, Berenstein A, TerBrugge K. Surgical neuroangiography: clinical and endovascular treatment aspects in adults, vol. 2.2. Berlin: Springer; 2004.

34

Case 35

João Xavier

References – 190

Brief history   28-year-old woman with cervicalgia.

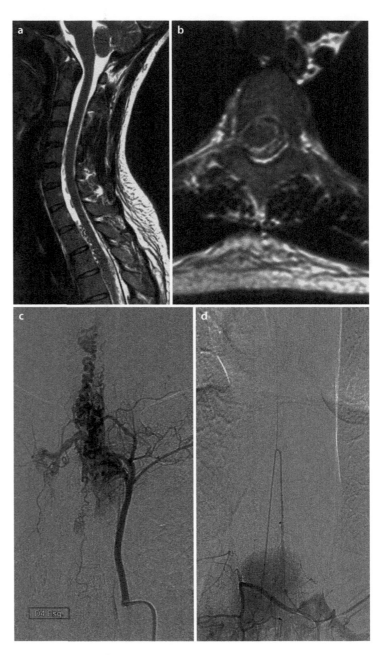

□ Fig. 35.1   a, b Sagittal and axial T2 weighted images, **c** and **d** DSA of left Th4 and right L1 segmental arteries

Case 35

? **Question 1: What is the diagnosis?**
(a) Dural arteriovenous fistula
(b) Spinal cord arteriovenous malformation
(c) Ependymoma
(d) High grade astrocytoma with intratumoral arteriovenous shunt
(e) Epidural arteriovenous shunt

? **Question 2: Image d shows**
(a) A minor arterial feeding branch of the hypervascularized lesion
(b) The anterior spinal artery
(c) The posterior spinal artery
(d) The Adamkiewicz artery
(e) One of the various posterior spinal arteries

? **Question 3: How should this patient be treated?**
(a) Wait and see
(b) Surgical excision of the lesion
(c) Endovascular exclusion with glue or Onyx
(d) Occlusion of left Th4 artery with coils, as near the lesion as possible
(e) Radiosurgery

Diagnosis   Spinal cord arteriovenous malformation

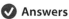 **Answers**

1. b.

Spinal arteriovenous lesions can be classified as arteriovenous malformations (AVM) or arteriovenous fistulae (AVF) depending on the presence or absence of a nidus between the arteries and the veins. Spinal cord AVMs represent 20–30% of spinal vascular malformations (SVM). They are high-flow lesions supplied by one or more branches of the anterior spinal artery (ASA) and/or posterior spinal arteries (PSA) with a discrete nidus [1]. In this case, main feeders arise from the anterior spinal artery (a thin ascending branch was seen in the early images of the Th4 run – ◘ Fig. 35.1c). Further classification on AVMs depends on their location. There are many vessels around the spinal cord, but they are mostly veins. In MR images, some vascular voids seem to be inside the spinal cord (see flow voids on ◘ Fig. 35.1a, b). Regardless, we cannot be sure if this is an intramedullary (also known as type II or glomus-type) AVM or a pial AVM. Spinal cord AVMs typically appear in childhood or early adulthood, with sudden onset of symptoms due to hemorrhage or compression-induced myelopathy [2]. In this patient, the diagnosis was incidental, after a cervical MR examination done for investigation of neck pain. Three years later, the patient is still asymptomatic.

2. d.

Of course, ◘ Fig. 35.1d is an image of a normal Adamkiewicz artery, with its typical hairpin form, feeding the ASA through ascending and descending branches [2].

3. a and c could be considered.

In an asymptomatic patient, therapeutic decision must be cautious, as any therapeutic option carries a high risk of spinal cord damage. If treatment is decided upon, endovascular nidus exclusion with liquid agents should be chosen. Feeder occlusion is not an option, as the malformation will recruit other feeders, surgery will damage the spinal cord, when looking for the shunt and radiosurgery cannot avoid having the spinal cord inside the radiation field.

References

1. Patsalides A, et al. Endovascular treatment of spinal arteriovenous lesions: beyond the dural fistula. AJNR Am J Neuroradiol. 2011;32:798–808.
2. Lasjaunias P, Berenstein A, ter Brugge KG. Surgical neuroangiography, vol. 1, 2. Berlin, Heidelberg: Springer-Verlag; 2004.

35

Case 36

João Xavier and José Eduardo Alves

References – 195

Brief history   A 12-year-old, previously healthy male with unremarkable family history was admitted to our institution with 3-day-long complaints of severe occipital headaches, nausea, vomiting and photophobia. For the past month, he had been experiencing right leg weakness with progressive gait disturbance and dysphagia.

Neurological examination showed pyramidal syndrome with slight right hemiparesis, tongue deviation towards the right, minimal right peripheral facial paresis and ataxia.

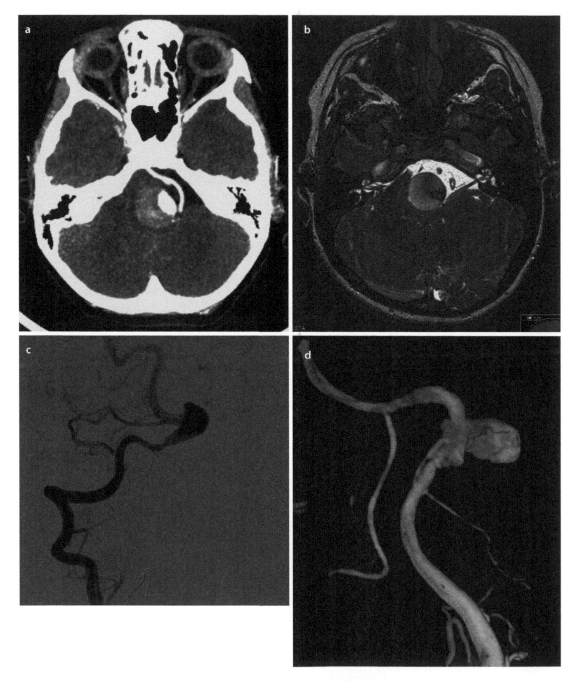

Fig. 36.1   **a** MIP axial CT scan with contrast medium; **b** axial T2 weighted image at IAC level; **c** DSA of right vertebral artery, frontal view; **d** DSA of right vertebral artery with 3D reconstruction

? **Question 1: What is the diagnosis?**
  (a) Saccular aneurysm of the right vertebral artery
  (b) Dissecting aneurysm of the right vertebral artery
  (c) Hypervascularised tumour of the brainstem
  (d) Arteriovenous malformation of the brainstem
  (e) Hydatid cyst with brain oedema

? **Question 2: What is the major risk to this patient?**
  (a) Subarachnoid haemorrhage
  (b) Intra-axial haemorrhage
  (c) Respiratory arrest
  (d) Tetraparesis
  (e) All the above

? **Question 3: How should this patient be treated?**
  (a) Antibiotic plus steroids
  (b) Surgical excision of the lesion
  (c) Endovascular exclusion with glue or Onyx
  (d) Occlusion of right vertebral artery
  (e) Lesion filling with coils and stenting

Diagnosis   Vertebral artery dissecting aneurysm

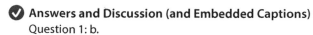 **Answers and Discussion (and Embedded Captions)**
Question 1: b.
Dissecting aneurysms are typically irregular and may be accompanied by pre-aneurysm vessel stenosis [1, 2], as can be seen on the DSA image (◘ Fig. 36.1c). 3D reconstruction (◘ Fig. 36.1d) shows a small side vessel that can result from a fenestration of the vertebral artery. This vessel was not amenable to micro-catheterisation at the time. CT and MR images (◘ Fig. 36.1a, b) show a partially thrombosed aneurysm, a huge mass effect on the brainstem with some oedema.
Question 2: e.
If the aneurysm continues to grow or if a rupture supervenes, all of these symptoms could occur. It is a high-risk situation.
Question 3: d.
The permeable part of the aneurysm must be excluded from the arterial circulation. After this, pulsatility over the brainstem should decrease and intramural/intra-luminal thrombus should also slowly decrease its volume. This aneurysm, as usually happens with dissecting aneurysms, does not have a defined neck. Putting coils inside it would probably lead to vessel occlusion. Besides, the aneurysm wall is weak and prone to rupture. In view of this, we planned to occlude the right vertebral artery, immediately proximal to the aneurysm. There was a major concern about this approach: the arterial supply to low cranial nerves and to spinal cord (note the thin feeder of anterior spinal artery in ◘ Fig. 36.1c, d). Due to this, the treatment was carried out under neurophysiological monitoring of motor-evoked potentials in the hypoglossus and accessory nerves and in the superior and inferior limbs, before every coil detachment. Absence of anterograde aneurysm filling was achieved, despite some residual retrograde filling from the left vertebral artery. It was decided to wait and see, in the hope that this residual filling would spontaneously disappear. The patient was discharged, without neurological deficits, but medium-term follow-up images showed that, although the total size of the aneurysm had decreased, the permeable part had become larger and once again contained anterograde filling through the side channel of the right vertebral artery, the diameter of which had increased (◘ Fig. 36.2a), becoming navigable. Through this, more coils were put inside the aneurysm, achieving its complete occlusion (and of the right vertebral artery) and decrease in size, as shown by a long-term follow-up image (◘ Fig. 36.2b, c).

36

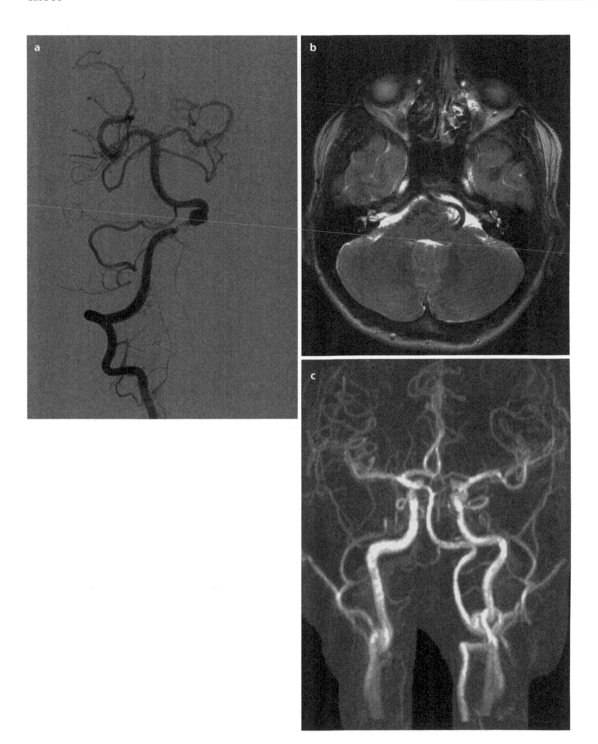

◘ Fig. 36.2 **a** DSA of right vertebral artery, frontal view, 16 months after first session; **b** axial T2 weighted image at IAC level, 1 year after second session (compare with ◘ Fig. 36.1b); **c** contrast medium MR-angiography, 1 year after second session

References

1. Kai Y, et al. Strategy for treating unruptured vertebral artery dissecting aneurysms. Neurosurgery. 2011;69:1085–92.
2. Wandong S, et al. Management of ruptured and unruptured intracranial vertebral artery dissecting aneurysms. J Clin Neurosci. 2011;18:1639–44.

Case 37

José Pedro Rocha Pereira, Viriato Alves, and Maria Goreti Sá

© Springer International Publishing AG 2018
J. Xavier et al. (eds.), *Diagnostic and Therapeutic Neuroradiology*,
https://doi.org/10.1007/978-3-319-61140-2_37

A 26-year-old, previously healthy female presented at the emergency department following an attempted suicide by drug overdose.

? Questions

1. What kind of arteriovenous shunt is represented, dural or pial?
2. Is it congenital or acquired?
3. Which are the main feeding arteries and the main venous drainage of the shunt?
4. How would you classify the shunt in the Cognard classification system?

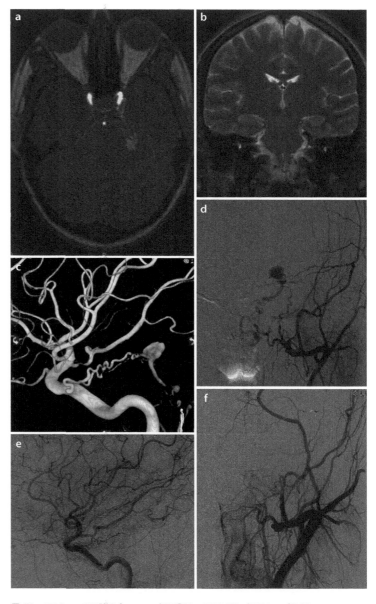

◘ Fig. 37.1   a 3D TOF; **b** coronal T2 TSE; **c** DSA 3D; **d** DSA; **e, f** DSA

Diagnosis   Tentorial dural fistula

✅ **Answers**
1. It is a tentorial marginal type dural fistula.
2. Dural fistulas are acquired arteriovenous shunts located within the dura of dural sinuses or, as in this case, in leptomeningeal veins, supplied by regional meningeal arteries.
3. The shunt is fed by the left marginal tentorial artery, which, in this case, has its origin in the left inferolateral and meningohypophyseal trunks (☐ Fig. 37.1a, c); it also has minor contributions from the left middle meningeal and accessory meningeal arteries (☐ Fig. 37.1d). The fistula point is in the left petrosal vein, which is ectasic and has two venous pouches, the largest one in the fistula point.
4. It is a type IV Cognard dural fistula.

The dural fistula was treated by endovascular approach, with onyx injection within the middle meningeal and accessory meningeal arteries. The shunt was excluded and the venous pouches of the petrosal vein completely deflated (☐ Fig. 37.1e, f).

37.1   Comments

Dural fistula etiology is not completely understood but the most accepted explanation regards venous thrombosis as a trigger factor for the development of the shunt. Apart from classifications based on anatomy, most classifications consider the drainage pattern, especially the presence of leptomeningeal venous reflux which poses a high risk of hemorrhage and/or venous congestion. Direct fistulas into leptomeningeal veins (extrasinusal fistulas – type III or IV according to the Cognard classification system) have a higher risk of cortical reflux and, if located in the posterior fossa, of perimedullary reflux – type V according to the Cognard classification system.

Tentorial dural fistulas are rare (accounting for 4–8% of all intracranial dural fistulas) [1] but represent one of the most life-threatening vascular lesions, because they drain exclusively into leptomeningeal veins. The reported occurrence of hemorrhage ranges from 60% to 74% [2], the highest value taking into account all locations of dural fistulas. Their arterial supply and venous drainage depend on the exact location of the shunt within the tentorium. In the marginal type (Picard's classification) [3], the shunt is located along the free edge of the tentorium, and the main feeder is the marginal tentorial artery.

References

1. Picard L, Bracard S, Islak C, Roy D, Moreno A, Marchal JC, Roland J. Dural fistulae of the tentorium cerebelli: radioanatomical, clinical and therapeutic considerations. J Neuroradiol. 1990;17(3):161–81.

2. Mitsuhashi Y, Aurboonyawat T, Pereira VM, Geibprasert S, Lasjaunias P. Dural arteriovenous fistulas draining into the petrosal vein or bridging vein of the medulla: possible homologs of spinal dural arteriovenous fistulas. J Neurosurg. 2009;111:889–99.
3. Cognard C, Gobin YP, Pierot L, et al. Cerebral dural arteriovenous fistulas: clinical and angiographic correlation with a revised classification of venous drainage. Radiology. 1995;194:671–80.

37

Case 38

Ricardo Almendra, Ana Graça Velon, and Inês Rego

© Springer International Publishing AG 2018
J. Xavier et al. (eds.), *Diagnostic and Therapeutic Neuroradiology*,
https://doi.org/10.1007/978-3-319-61140-2_38

A 52-year-old woman was admitted to the emergency department with nausea and vomiting lasting 5 h, right-sided decreased muscle strength, and liquid dysphagia. Neurological examination revealed a left-beating nystagmus, mild dysarthria, diminished gag reflex, right hemiparesis grade 3/5 mRC, right hemiataxia, left hemihypo-esthesia, and right Babinski sign (NIHSS 8).

❓ Questions

1. What are the findings?
2. Is there an explanation for the ipsilateral hemiparesis?
3. What is the name of the condition with these clinical and imagiological findings?

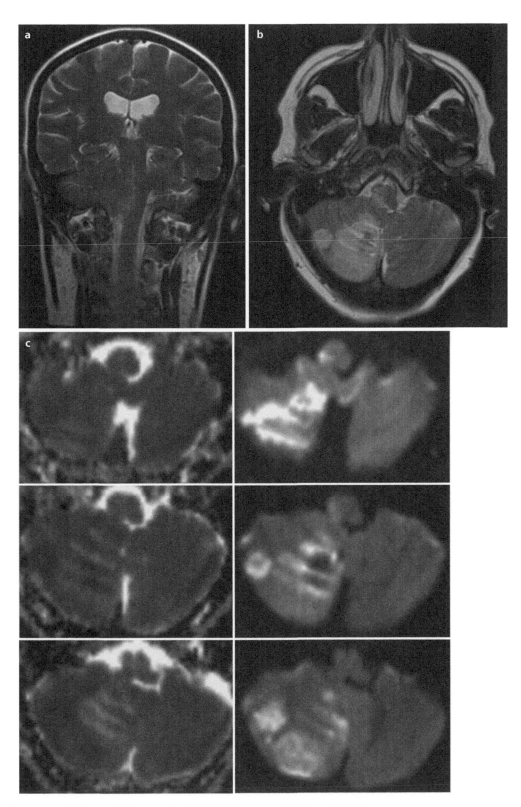

Diagnosis   Opalski syndrome

✓ **Answers to Questions**

1. T2 hyperintensity of the right medullary and right cerebellar lesions (◘ Fig. 38.1a, b), presenting with slight mass effect and with restricted diffusion in the same region (◘ Fig. 38.1c), corresponds to an acute ischemic stroke in the PICA territory.
2. The ischemic lesion extends inferiorly and affects the corticospinal tract caudal to the pyramidal decussation (◘ Fig. 38.1a).
3. The lateral medullary stroke, also named Wallenberg syndrome, can, in rare cases, be accompanied with ipsilateral hemiparesis. This clinical syndrome was named Opalski syndrome after its description in 1946 [1].

38.1 Comments

The posterior inferior cerebellar artery is responsible for the supply of the entire lateral medullary region between the medullary pyramids and the fasciculus cuneatus at the caudal medullary level. The classic PICA stroke presents as Wallenberg syndrome. When the lesion is caudal, it can involve the corticospinal tract after pyramidal decussation causing an ipsilateral hemiparesis. Sometimes cerebellar PICA territory can also be included [2].

References

1. Opalski A. Un nouveau syndrome sous-bulbaire: syndrome partiel de l'artère vertébro-spinale postérieur. Paris Med. 1946;1:214–20.
2. Kumral E, Kisabay A, Atac C, Calli C, Yunten N. Spectrum of the posterior inferior cerebellar artery territory infarcts. Clinical-diffusion-weighted imaging correlates. Cerebrovasc Dis. 2005;20:370–80.

Case 39

Cláudia Pereira

© Springer International Publishing AG 2018
J. Xavier et al. (eds.), *Diagnostic and Therapeutic Neuroradiology*,
https://doi.org/10.1007/978-3-319-61140-2_39

A 82-year-old diabetic man, 6 h post cardiopulmonary arrest of unknown cause.

? Questions

1. What are the imaging findings?
2. What is your main differential diagnosis?
3. What is the «reversal sign»?

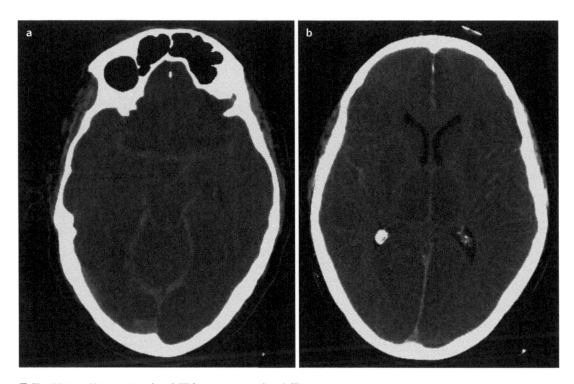

◻ Fig. 39.1   a Non-contrast head CT, **b** non-contrast head CT

Diagnosis   Hypoxic-ischaemic encephalopathy

✅ Answers

1. Imaging findings include increased density of the basal cisterns, falx, tentorium and cerebral sulci (◨ Fig. 39.1a), low-density lesions in the grey matter and cerebral oedema with sulci effacement (◨ Fig. 39.1b).
2. Hypoxic-ischaemic encephalopathy or subarachnoid haemorrhage.
3. The reversal sign is seen on unenhanced computed tomographic (CT) images of the brain as an inversion of the normal attenuation relationship between grey and white matter; grey matter presents relatively lower density than adjacent white matter. The reversal sign is associated with a poor prognosis and indicates irreversible brain damage [3].

39.1   Comments

Hypoxic-ischaemic encephalopathy results from a global insult due to profound loss of cerebral blood supply or hypoxia, despite adequate perfusion.

In adults, the most commonly related clinical events are cardiopulmonary arrest, severe hypotension or hypertension, trauma and venous sinus thrombosis [1].

There is usually bilateral and symmetric damage and cortical and deep grey matter are more frequently affected as neurons are more vulnerable to hypoxia than oligodendroglia or astrocytes.

CT abnormalities in the acute and subacute phases are usually seen only in severe cases and include pseudo-subarachnoid haemorrhage (erroneous appearance of subarachnoid haemorrhage, with false increased density of the basal cisterns, sulci, falx and tentorium) [2], diffuse cerebral oedema with effacement of the CSF-containing spaces, loss of grey/white matter differentiation, low-density lesions in the basal ganglia with the «reversal sign» [3] and the white cerebellum sign (preserved attenuation in the cerebellum and brainstem, which appear relatively hyperdense when compared to the diffuse low attenuation of cerebral hemispheres due to oedema).

References

1. Gutierrez L, Rovira A, Portela L, Leite C, Lucato L. CT and MR in non-neonatal hypoxic-ischemic encephalopathy: radiological findings with pathophysiological correlations. Neuroradiology. 2010;52:949–76.
2. Given CA 2nd, Burdette JH, Elster AD, Williams DW 3rd. Pseudo-subarachnoid hemorrhage: a potential imaging pitfall associated with diffuse cerebral edema. AJNR Am J Neuroradiol. 2003;24(2):254–6.
3. Kavanagh EC. The reversal sign. Radiology. 2007;245(3):914–5.

Degenerative Diseases

Contents

Case 40

Pedro Pinto

© Springer International Publishing AG 2018
J. Xavier et al. (eds.), *Diagnostic and Therapeutic Neuroradiology*,
https://doi.org/10.1007/978-3-319-61140-2_40

A 57-year-old man with progressive onset of difficulty in driving and manual procedures and superior limb tremor. The patient had numerous appointments with opticians and ophthalmologists due to difficulty in locating and perceiving objects. Apathy and depression were also main clinical features; however, anxiety, aggression/agitation, psychosis, and memory deficits were not found. The neurological exam did not find focal deficits, but the patient presented with apraxia, visual agnosia, and a more pronounced superior limb tremor on the right side.

? Questions

1. What are the main imaging features?
2. Which of these three MRI sequences is the best to evaluate global cortical atrophy?
3. What are the main differential diagnoses?

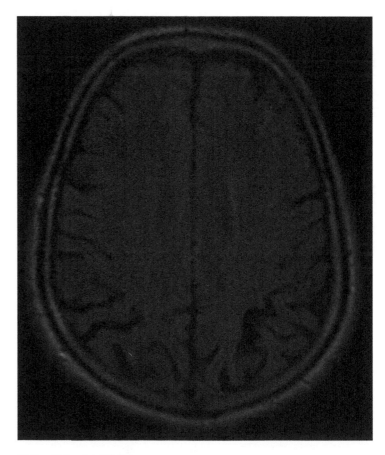

◻ **Fig. 40.1**   Axial FLAIR

Case 40

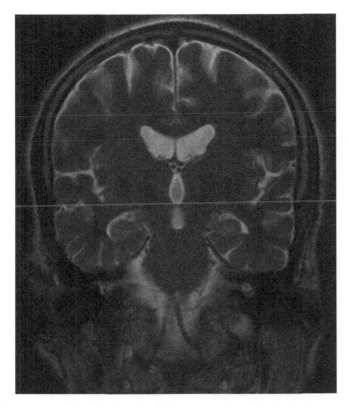

■ Fig. 40.2 Coronal T2-WI

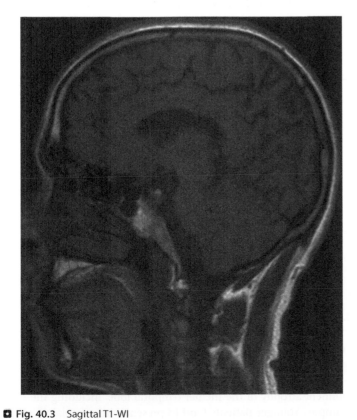

■ Fig. 40.3 Sagittal T1-WI

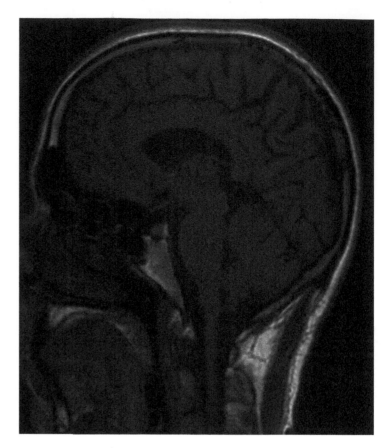

◘ **Fig. 40.4** Coronal T2-WI

Diagnosis   Early-onset Alzheimer disease

✔ **Answers to the Questions**

1. Slight global cortical atrophy with involvement of bilateral parietal lobes (◘ Figs. 40.1, 40.2, and 40.3), especially the precuneus regions between the parieto-occipital sulci and the pars marginalis of the cingulate sulcus, sparing the medial temporal lobes (◘ Fig. 40.4)
2. Fluid-attenuated inversion recovery (FLAIR) sequence (◘ Fig. 40.1)
3. Vascular dementia, frontotemporal dementia, corticobasal degeneration syndrome, and dementia with Lewy bodies

40

40.1 **Comments**

In elderly patients AD is usually characterized by insidious onset of cognitive decline, starting with memory impairment and followed by global cognitive decline. Imaging studies show global atrophy with prominent atrophy of the medial temporal lobe, including the hippocampus. Younger patients tend to present with complaints other than memory impairment, such as visuospatial problems and apraxia. Posterior atrophy is more prevalent in this setting, resulting in atrophy of either the parietal lobe or the precuneus, including the posterior cingulate [1]. The precuneus is located in the medial aspect of the posterior parietal lobe, and its borders are the parieto-occipital sulcus posteriorly and the marginal ramus (pars marginalis) of the cingulate sulcus anteriorly. Precuneus is best appreciated on midsagittal section. The association with ApoE4 genotype seen with amnestic Alzheimer's disease might not be observed in patients with posterior cortical atrophy, hinting at neurobiological differences between these groups of patients [2].

References

1. Karas G, et al. Precuneus atrophy in early-onset Alzheimer's disease: a morphometric structural MRI study. Neuroradiology. 2007;49:967–76.
2. Rossor M, et al. The diagnosis of young-onset dementia. Lancet Neurol. 2010;9(8):793–806.

Case 41

Luís Botelho, Carla Silva, Nuno Vila-Chã, Alexandre Mendes, and António Verdelho

© Springer International Publishing AG 2018
J. Xavier et al. (eds.), *Diagnostic and Therapeutic Neuroradiology*,
https://doi.org/10.1007/978-3-319-61140-2_41

41.1 History

A 67-year-old male with progressive intention tremor which started 15 years ago, now presenting severe disability, worse in the right hand, with limited response to pharmacological therapy.

❓ Questions

1. What kind of procedure is displayed in the images?
2. Which specific nucleus is targeted within the thalamus for optimal therapeutic results?
3. The targeted nucleus has somatotopic organisation. In the case of tremor that predominantly involves the upper limb, should the target be placed more laterally or medially in contrast to a lower limb preference?

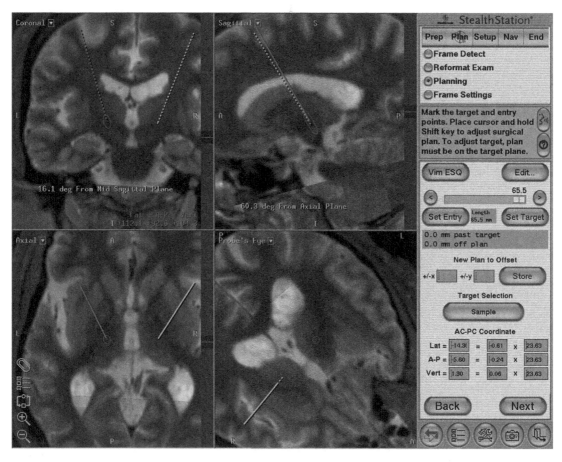

▢ **Fig. 41.1**   3T MR, target planning on T2 WAIR images

Case 41

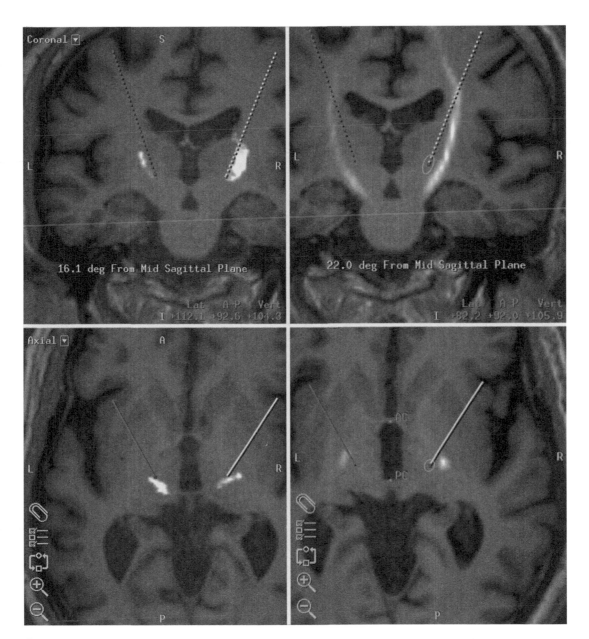

Fig. 41.2 T1 fused with motor thalamus parcellations (*left*) and with the corticospinal tracts (*right*)

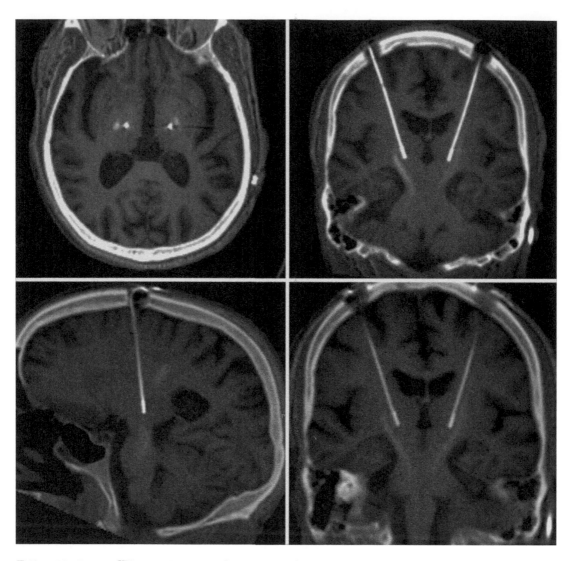

◘ Fig. 41.3 Post-op CT in co-registration with pre-op MR T1 images with corticospinal tracts

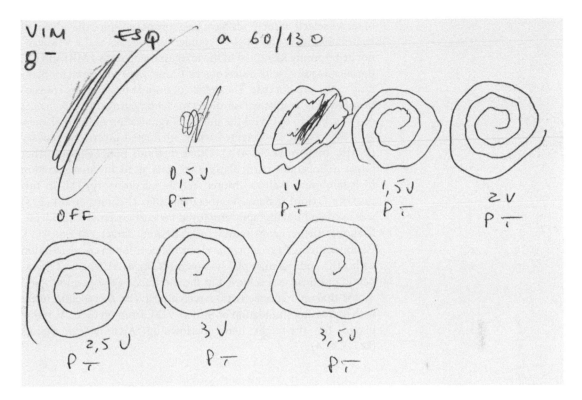

◘ Fig. 41.4 Patient drawings with the right hand: Off stimulation (*left upper corner*) and with increasing voltage stimulation

Diagnosis Essential tremor

✓ **Answers**
1. Deep brain stimulation surgery.
2. Thalamic ventralis intermedius (VIM) nucleus (Hassler terminology).
3. The target should be more medially adjusted for the upper limb vs the lower limb. In the somatotopic organisation of the VIM, the head is located in a more medial position, the upper limb in an intermediate position and the lower limb laterally next to the posterior limb of the internal capsule.

41.2 **Comments**

Essential tremor is regarded as the most common movement disorder. It has heterogeneous presentation with mild forms that do not require treatment and more severe cases that are usually manageable with pharmacological therapy. Patients having relentless progression of tremor with increased disability refractory to pharmacological treatment may benefit from deep brain stimulation surgery. This accurate stereotactic procedure requires image planning combined with intraoperative neurophysiology recording and stimulation to determine the ideal electrode placement with maximum benefit while minimising potential side effects. A variety of target selection methods have been proposed since the advent of ventriculography and MRI/CT-guided approaches as the VIM cannot be promptly identified in the images. Preoperative MRI and CT, the later acquired with a stereotactic frame, were employed for planning in the present case. The detail commonly provided by conventional MRI is insufficient for direct nuclei targeting. MRI sequences can be adjusted to reveal the internal organisation of the thalamus, as is the case of T2-weighted white attenuated inversion recovery (WAIR) images (◘ Fig. 41.1). Other methods may help in further target delineation, particularly atlas data used in co-registration (Schaltenbrand-Wahren, Morel, Yelnik, Chakravarty) [1]. In this case the Oxford thalamic connectivity atlas (Behrens et al.) [2, 3] was used and tractography employed for corticospinal tract identification, further constraining the desired target (◘ Fig. 41.2). Postoperative CT revealing the electrode position in co-registration with MRI and tractography is shown (◘ Fig. 41.3). The best therapeutic response was achieved at the interface of the premotor and motor thalamic connectivity parcellations. The therapeutic result with increasing stimulation of the left VIM, from off to 3.5 V, is displayed for the right hand performing Archimedean spirals (◘ Fig. 41.4).

References

1. Bardinet E, Belaid H, Grabli D, Welter M-L, Vidal SF, Galanaud D, et al. Thalamic stimulation for tremor: can target determination be improved? Mov Disord. 2011;26(2):307–12.
2. Behrens TEJ, Johansen-Berg H, Woolrich MW, Smith SM, Wheeler-Kingshott CAM, Boulby PA, et al. Non-invasive mapping of connections between human thalamus and cortex using diffusion imaging. Nat Neurosci. 2003;6(7):750–7.
3. Pouratian N, Zheng Z, Bari AA, Behnke E, Jeff Elias W, DeSalles AAF. Multi-institutional evaluation of deep brain stimulation targeting using probabilistic connectivity-based thalamic segmentation. J Neurosurg. 2011;115(5): 995–1004.

Case 42

Cristina Ramos

© Springer International Publishing AG 2018
J. Xavier et al. (eds.), *Diagnostic and Therapeutic Neuroradiology*,
https://doi.org/10.1007/978-3-319-61140-2_42

A 36-year-old patient. Tetrapyramidal syndrome with paresis, hyperreflexia and tongue atrophy. 2.5 years of evolution.

? Questions
1. What are the findings on these MR images?
2. What are the main clinical hallmarks of this entity?
3. Is there an association with other pathologies?

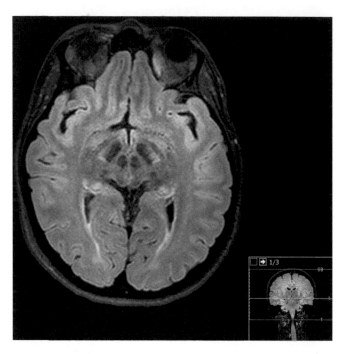

◼ Fig. 42.1   Axial FLAIR

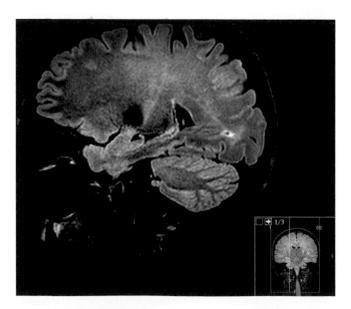

◼ Fig. 42.2   Sagittal FLAIR

42

Case 42

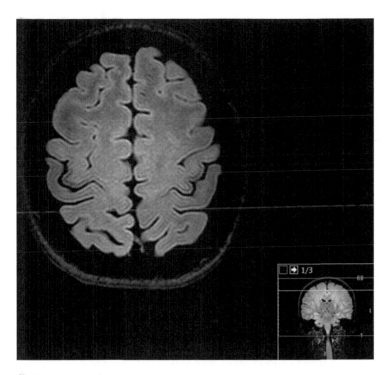

Fig. 42.3 Axial FLAIR

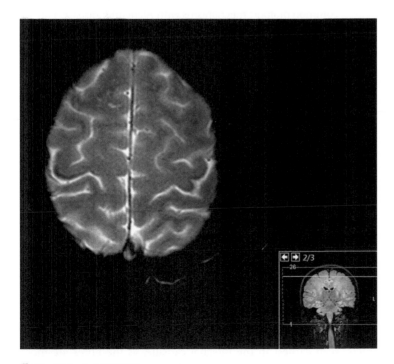

Fig. 42.4 Axial T2 GRE

Diagnosis   Motor neuron disease – amyotrophic lateral sclerosis

✅ **Answers to Questions**

1. T2 and FLAIR hyperintensity in corticospinal tracts (◾ Figs. 42.1 and 42.2) (specificity <70% and sensitivity <40%), seen on cerebral peduncles (◾ Fig. 42.1) and in the posterior limb of the internal capsule (◾ Fig. 42.2); T2* (◾ Fig. 42.4) and FLAIR (◾ Fig. 42.3) hypointensity on the cortical ribbon of the motor cortex represents iron deposition [3].

2. Clinical hallmarks of this disease include involvement of upper and lower motor neurons, with clinical signs of decreased motor strength, hyperreflexia, muscle atrophy and fasciculations, especially involving the muscles of the face, tongue and hands, with progressive spread of signs to other regions. Although there is progressive loss of motor strength, there is preservation of sensory and intellectual status [1, 2].

3. The cause of amyotrophic lateral sclerosis (ALS) is unknown, although some environmental causes have been implicated, such as smoking. Family history of the disease is positive in about 5–10% of patients, and twin studies show a genetic contribution, with heritability of about 61%. In some cases, ALS overlaps clinically, pathologically and biologically with frontotemporal dementia, and it may share common biologic mechanisms with Alzheimer disease, Parkinson disease and other neurodegenerative diseases [2].

42.1 Comments

Amyotrophic lateral sclerosis (ALS) is the most common degenerative disease of the motor neuron system. ALS is a relentlessly progressive neurological disorder characterised by the death of upper motor neurons (Betz cells in the cortex) and anterior horn cells of the spinal cord with secondary Wallerian degeneration.

Both upper and lower motor neurons are affected. Loss of lower motor neurons leads to progressive muscle weakness with atrophy, fasciculations, loss of reflexes and muscle tone. Loss of corticospinal upper motor neurons usually leads to milder weakness associated with spasticity and brisk reflexes. There is a progressive loss of motor strength with preservation of sensory and intellectual functions.

Approximately 15% of patients with ALS also meet criteria for frontotemporal dementia (FTD) [1, 2].

The neuroimaging of this entity is characteristic. The earliest MR manifestation is hyperintensity on T2WI in the corticospinal tracts, seen earliest in the internal capsule, as the fibres are most concentrated here. Eventually, the entire tract from the motor strip to the spinal cord is affected, showing increased T2 signal and volume loss. Iron deposition in the cortex is demonstrated as hypointensity, seen on T2 but most evident on T2*-weighted sequences [3].

ALS typically progresses to death in 2–6 years, usually from respiratory complications [1, 2].

42

References

1. Brooks BR, Miller RG, Swash M, Munsat TL. El Escorial revisited: revised criteria for the diagnosis of amyotrophic lateral sclerosis. Amyotroph Lateral Scler Other Motor Neuron Disord. 2000;1(5):293–9.
2. Hardiman O, van den Berg LH, Kiernan MC. Clinical diagnosis and management of amyotrophic lateral sclerosis. Nat Rev Neurol. 2011;7(11):639–49.
3. Cheung G, Gawel MJ, Cooper PW, et al. Amyotrophic lateral sclerosis: correlation of clinical and MR imaging findings. Radiology. 1995;194(1):263–70.

Case 43

Cristina Ramos

© Springer International Publishing AG 2018
J. Xavier et al. (eds.), *Diagnostic and Therapeutic Neuroradiology*,
https://doi.org/10.1007/978-3-319-61140-2_43

A 8-year-old patient, with a history of Rasmussen encephalitis, left hemiparesis, hyperreflexia and Babinski sign.

❓ Questions

1. What are the findings on these MR images?
2. What is the MRI sequence and interpretation of the bottom row images?
3. In what pathologies can this occur?

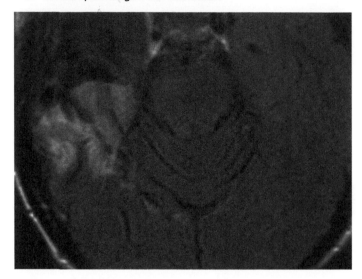

◘ Fig. 43.1   Axial FLAIR

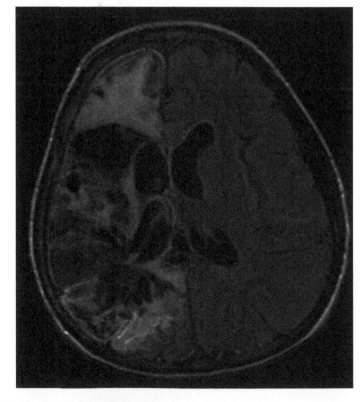

◘ Fig. 43.2   Axial FLAIR

43

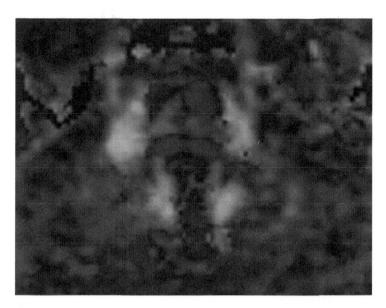

Fig. 43.3 Axial DTI – FA/colour map

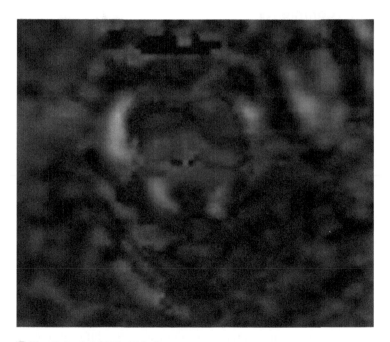

Fig. 43.4 Axial DTI – FA/colour map

Diagnosis   Wallerian degeneration of corticospinal tract

✅ Answers to Questions

1. Large right hemispheric destructive lesion with no arterial territory, due to sequelae of Rasmussen encephalitis (▣ Fig. 43.2). Note also the FLAIR hyperintensity on the right basis pontis (▣ Fig. 43.1), located far away from the supratentorial lesion, suggestive of Wallerian degeneration (WD) of the corticospinal tract (CST).
2. The bottom row images (▣ Figs. 43.3 and 43.4) are the FA/colour maps of DTI sequence, showing striking asymmetry between CST, with lower FA on the right side, consistent with anatomic images that suggest WD.
3. This can occur with different lesions which affect the supratentorial CST, including stroke, haemorrhage, neurodegenerative diseases such as motor neuron disease and Rasmussen encephalitis (▣ Fig. 43.2), which is the case of our patient.

43.1 Comments

Wallerian degeneration (WD) consists of the anterograde degeneration of axons and their myelin sheaths after proximal axonal or cell body injury from numerous causes, including stroke, inflammatory and neurodegenerative diseases, where the extent of WD in the CST is one of the major determinants of motor deficit. Severe WD in the CST distal to a supratentorial infarct in the acute stage has been considered a predictor of worse motor outcome [2].

Many studies have reported hyperintensity on T2-weighted or diffusion-weighted imaging along the affected CST weeks or months after stroke, and this finding correlates well with persistent functional disability. However, on conventional MR imaging, these findings are usually subtle and can be difficult to detect in the first few weeks. Additionally, the extent of WD is difficult to quantify on conventional MR imaging and is not consistent in all patients with motor deficit.

DTI provides information on the predominant direction and coherence of tissue water diffusion. The degree of anisotropy depends on the level of organisation and integrity of the white matter tract and on the degree of freedom of water diffusion movements by oriented axonal membranes and myelin sheaths. Reduced anisotropy along the CST far away from a brain lesion has been interpreted as WD, even when CST in these areas appeared normal on conventional MR imaging [1, 2].

Signal-intensity abnormalities related to WD are generally not detected until 4 weeks after stroke; after this time the main finding is a hyperintensity along the affected tracts on DWI and T2-weighted images. Even in patients with motor deficits who do not have signal-intensity abnormalities on conventional MR imaging, there are differences in anisotropy, with decreased FA values on the affected side of the CST. Additionally, the signal-intensity change in the affected

43

CST is strongly associated with lower FA indexes. These findings suggest that DTI is more sensitive in detecting tissue changes of WD than conventional MR imaging and can give additional information in terms of prognosis [1, 2].

References

1. Thomalla G, Glauche V, Weiller C, et al. Time course of wallerian degeneration after ischaemic stroke revealed by diffusion tensor imaging. J Neurol Neurosurg Psychiatry. 2005;76:266–8.
2. Puig J, Pedraza S, Blasco G, Daunis-I-Estadella J, Prats A, Prados F, et al. Wallerian degeneration in the corticospinal tract evaluated by diffusion tensor imaging correlates with motor deficit 30 days after middle cerebral artery ischemic stroke. AJNR Am J Neuroradiol. 2010;31:1324–30.

Case 44

Ricardo Martins and José Eduardo Alves

© Springer International Publishing AG 2018
J. Xavier et al. (eds.), *Diagnostic and Therapeutic Neuroradiology*,
https://doi.org/10.1007/978-3-319-61140-2_44

An 84-year-old, partially dependent woman, presented with a progressive course of visual hallucinations and fluctuating confusional state for 2 months. One week prior to admission, she was found lying in bed, disoriented, with incoherent speech and refusing food and rapidly evolved with deterioration of conscience. On hospital admission, she was in a comatose state, severely dehydrated and emaciated. The initial workup showed no signs of infection.

? Questions

1. What bulbar structures are hyperintense in ☉ Fig. 44.1c (black arrows)?
2. What other supratentorial structures would one expect to be typically involved in this disorder?
3. What blood analysis could confirm the most likely diagnosis?

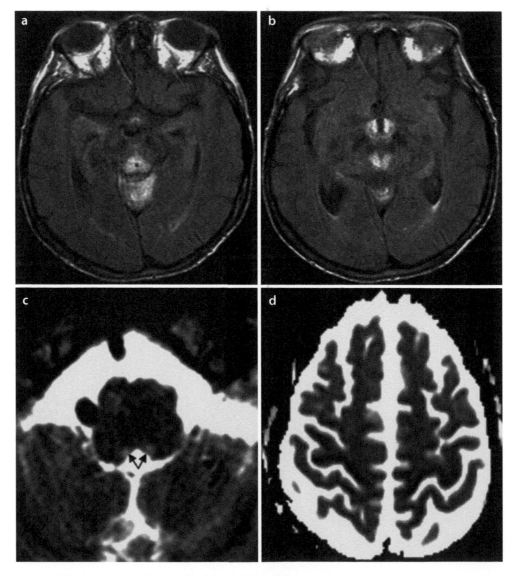

☉ **Fig. 44.1**   MRI **a, b** axial T2 FLAIR, **c** axial T2 TSE and **d** ADC map

Diagnosis   Wernicke's encephalopathy

 Answers
1. The hypoglossal nuclei
2. Dorsomedial thalami
3. Blood thiamine concentration

44.1 Comments

Wernicke's encephalopathy is an acute neurological disorder, resulting from thiamine (vitamin B1) deficiency which, when untreated, produces severe deficits, with progression to coma and even death. The prognosis strongly relies on early recognition and thiamine supplementation. Neuroimaging plays a central role in the diagnosis of Wernicke's encephalopathy, particularly in patients with no history of alcohol abuse or presenting with atypical clinical manifestations. MRI can show both *typical*, symmetric T2 hyperintensity in the dorsomedial thalami, tectal plate, periaqueductal area and mammillary bodies (◘ Fig. 44.1a, b), and *atypical*, T2 hyperintense lesions in the cerebellum, cerebellar vermis, cranial nerve nuclei (◘ Fig. 44.1c) and cerebral cortex, features, the latter being characteristic of non-alcoholic patients [1]. In the acute phase, affected regions may show restricted diffusion (◘ Fig. 44.1d) and contrast enhancement [2].

References

1. Zuccoli G, et al. Neuroimaging findings in acute Wernicke's encephalopathy: review of the literature. AJR. 2009;192:501–8.
2. Manzo G, et al. MR imaging findings in alcoholic and nonalcoholic acute Wernicke's encephalopathy: a review. Biomed Res Int. 2014;2014:503–96.

Case 45

Sofia Reimão, Pedro Viana, and Carla Guerreiro

© Springer International Publishing AG 2018
J. Xavier et al. (eds.), *Diagnostic and Therapeutic Neuroradiology*,
https://doi.org/10.1007/978-3-319-61140-2_45

A 63-year-old woman with parkinsonic symptoms, poorly responsive to levodopa/carbidopa.

? Questions

1. What are the imaging findings?
2. Are these findings compatible with the diagnosis of Parkinson's disease?
3. Can these imaging findings aid in the diagnosis?

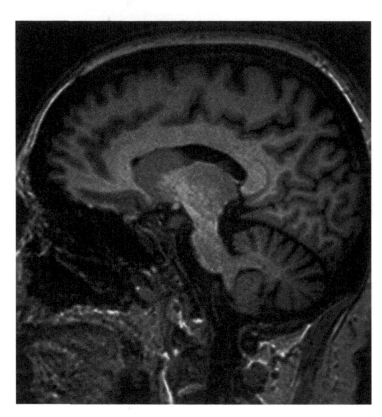

◘ **Fig. 45.1** Sagittal T1

Case 45

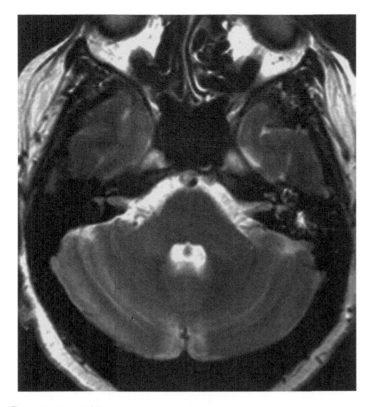

Fig. 45.2 Axial T2

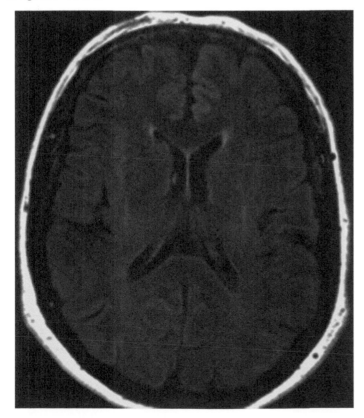

Fig. 45.3 Axial FLAIR

45

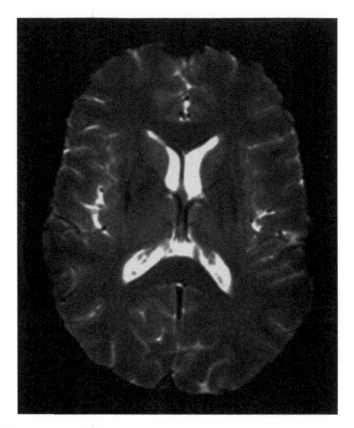

Fig. 45.4 Axial T2*

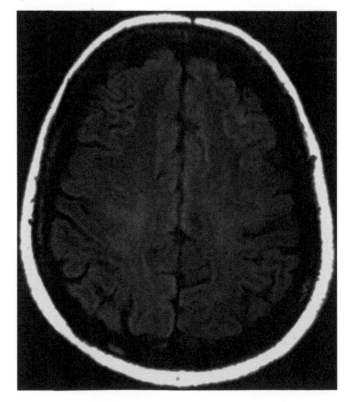

Fig. 45.5 Axial FLAIR

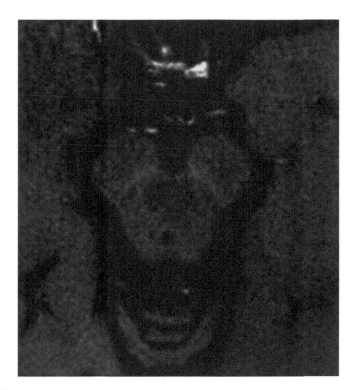

⬛ Fig. 45.6 Axial T1

Diagnosis Multiple system atrophy - parkinsonian type (MSA-P)

✅ **Answers to Questions**
1. Brain MRI sagittal T1- and axial T2-weighted images show dimensional reduction of the pons and the middle cerebellar peduncles (⬛ Figs. 45.1 and 45.2), with discrete T2 hyperintensity in the middle cerebellar peduncles (⬛ Fig. 45.2). Bilateral putaminal dorsolateral changes are visible on axial FLAIR (⬛ Fig. 45.3), with a «slit-like» marginal T2-hyperintensity rim, and on axial T2* (⬛ Fig. 45.4), showing dorsolateral putaminal hypointensity, corresponding to increased iron deposition. Axial FLAIR image (⬛ Fig. 45.5) shows bilateral hyperintensity in subcortical precentral gyrus. The normal *substantia nigra* T1-high signal corresponding to neuromelanin is preserved (⬛ Fig. 45.6).
2. Neuromelanin sensitive MR imaging has been used in the diagnosis and differential diagnosis of Parkinson's disease (PD), showing marked reduction of neuromelanin signal in the *substantia nigra* and *locus coeruleus,* even in early disease stages of PD. In this case, the neuromelanin signal in the substantia nigra and *locus coeruleus* is preserved, which is not suggestive of PD.
3. The diagnosis of Parkinson's disease can be challenging, particularly in early stages. In atypical/uncertain cases, the exclusive use of clinical criteria for diagnosis can have a high rate of misdiagnosis, even if performed by movement

disorders-specialized neurologists. Imaging can help in the differential diagnosis of atypical parkinsonian syndromes. The imaging findings in this case, with reduction of the middle cerebellar peduncles and putaminal signal changes, associated with motor cortex and subcortical alterations, are suggestive of the diagnosis of MSA-P. Atypical parkinsonian syndromes show a poor response to dopamine and have, in general, a worse prognosis than Parkinson's disease and so, when there is a clinical suspicion of these syndromes, MR imaging can be of great value in individual patient management.

45.1 Comments

Multiple system atrophy (MSA) is an idiopathic progressive neurodegenerative disorder, characterized clinically by autonomic dysfunction (mandatory for diagnosis), and a combination of parkinsonism, cerebellar dysfunction, and pyramidal tract dysfunction. Further classification is based on the predominant motor manifestation: MSA-P where parkinsonian features predominate and MSA-C where cerebellar features predominate.

In clinical practice, MSA-P can be misdiagnosed as idiopathic Parkinson's disease (PD), especially during the early stages. The revised consensus criteria for the diagnosis of MSA have included, not only clinical features but also magnetic resonance imaging (MRI) as supporting evidence for the diagnosis.

In patients with MSA-P, there is putaminal atrophy and abnormal T2-weighted hypointensity of the posterolateral putamen due to the susceptibility effect of iron [1]. It often progresses to the point that the putamen becomes darker than the *globus pallidus* («signal inversion»). Gliosis and neuronal degeneration is considered as a possible cause of the T2 hyperintensity seen along the lateral margins of the putamen. Neuromelanin sensitive MR images may help to differentiate MSA from PD [2].

In MSA-C, the neuronal degeneration is more pronounced in the pons, cerebellum, and inferior olives, and MRI scans show a significant atrophy of both the pons and the cerebellum. Typical cruciform hyperintensities in the pons on axial T2 are known as the «hot cross bun» sign (not pictured in this case).

Signs of pyramidal tract degeneration detected by MRI were only recently demonstrated in MSA cases [3].

References

1. Chandran V, Stoessl AJ. Imaging in multiple system atrophy. Neurol Clin Neurosci. 2014;2(6):178–87.
2. Reimão S, Pita Lobo P, Neutel D, Correia Guedes L, Coelho M, Rosa MM, et al. Substantia nigra neuromelanin magnetic resonance imaging in de novo Parkinson's disease patients. Eur J Neurol. 2015;22:540–6.
3. da Rocha AJ, Maia A, da Silva CJ, Braga F, Ferreira N, Barsottini O, et al. Pyramidal tract degeneration in multiple system atrophy: the relevance of magnetization transfer imaging. Mov Disord. 2007;22(2):238–43.

Spine

Contents

Case 46

Alexandra C. Lopes, José Pedro R. Pereira, and Cristina Ramos

© Springer International Publishing AG 2018
J. Xavier et al. (eds.), *Diagnostic and Therapeutic Neuroradiology*,
https://doi.org/10.1007/978-3-319-61140-2_46

46.1 Clinical Information

A 50-year-old female with *torticollis*, cervical stiffness, left cervico-brachialgia and odynophagia. Laboratory tests were not performed.

? Questions

1. Name the Findings.
2. Which differential diagnosis should be considered?
3. What is the aetiopathogeny?

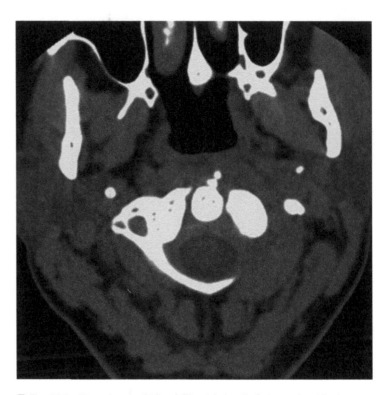

◻ Fig. 46.1 Non-contrast C1 level CT, axial view (soft tissue algorithm)

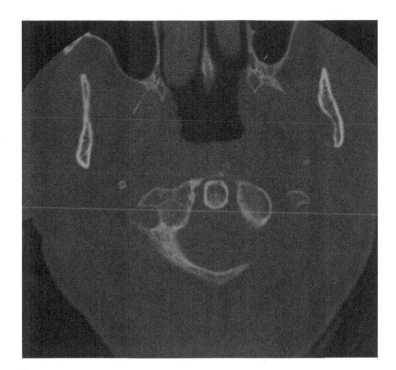

Fig. 46.2 Non-contrast C1 level CT, axial view (bone algorithm)

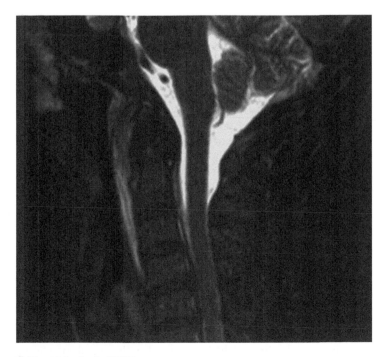

Fig. 46.3 Sagital T2WI

46

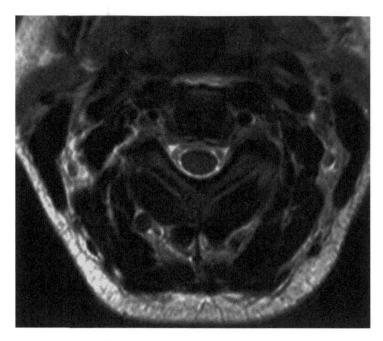

Fig. 46.4 Axial T2WI

Diagnosis Acute calcific tendinitis of the longus colli muscle

✔ Answers

1. Posterior nasopharyngeal wall thickening (◘ Fig. 46.1) and midline small prevertebral calcifications (◘ Fig. 46.2) on CT images; extensive effusion in the retropharyngeal space (◘ Figs. 46.3 and 46.4) on MRI
2. Retropharyngeal infection; post-traumatic oedema
3. Secondary inflammatory process due to the deposition of calcium hydroxyapatite in the superior oblique tendon fibres of the longus colli muscle(s)

46.2 Comments

The bilateral longus colli muscles, along with the longus capitis muscles, make up the bulk of the prevertebral space [2]. The retropharyngeal space is a deep neck space that contains fat and lymph nodes [2].

Pathologic conditions involving the prevertebral space are usually secondary to primary diseases affecting the spine (infections or tumour). Primary prevertebral disease is quite uncommon. The retropharyngeal space might be involved with several infections; this space may present oedema either after radiation therapy or after jugular vein resection.

Acute calcified longus colli tendinitis (ACLCT) was first described by Hartley in 1964. Posteriorly, in 1994, it was shown by Ring and colleagues to be an inflammatory condition secondary to the deposition of calcium hydroxyapatite in the tendon muscle fibres. It is thought to be a rare pathologic entity (age-matched incidence of 1.31 per 100.000 person-years, Horowitz et al.) and typically starts with neck pain, followed by stiffness of the neck and odynophagia. Laboratory studies are usually within normal limits.

Awareness of its principle imagiologic findings: thickening of prevertebral soft tissues and focal calcifications within the longus colli muscle tendon (usually at C1-C2 level) allows for an earlier diagnosis and proper treatment and thus prevents unnecessary invasive diagnostic procedures [1].

ACLCT is usually a self-limiting condition that tends to resolve itself after 1–3 weeks [1]. Symptoms can be relieved with a short course of non-steroidal anti-inflammatory medication and conservative treatment.

References

1. Ade S, Tunguturi A, Mitchell A. Acute calcific longus colli tendinitis: an underdiagnosed cause of neck pain and dysphagia. Neurol Bull. 2013;5. https://doi.org/10.7191/neurol_bull.2013.1043.
2. Eastwood JD, Hudgins PA, Malone D. Retropharyngeal effusion in acute calcific Prevertebral tendinitis: diagnosis with CT and MR imaging. AJNR Am J Neuroradiol. 1998;19:1789–92.

Case 47

Marta Rodrigues and Joana Nunes

© Springer International Publishing AG 2018
J. Xavier et al. (eds.), *Diagnostic and Therapeutic Neuroradiology*,
https://doi.org/10.1007/978-3-319-61140-2_47

47

A 4-year-old boy was taken to the emergency service with pain in the lumbar region and thighs, gait imbalance and reluctance to walk, of approximately 3 weeks duration. On physical examination he had a defensive gait caused by pain and rotation of the left inferior limb. No other signs or symptoms were present, including fever. The child had no relevant clinical background (◘ Figs. 47.1, 47.2, 47.3 and 47.4).

❓ Questions

1. What are the imaging findings?
2. What are the possible differential diagnoses?
3. Which other relevant results of additional investigation are present?

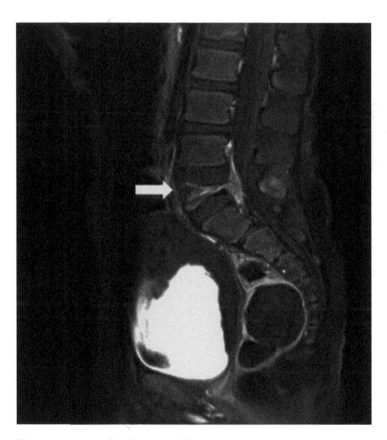

◘ Fig. 47.1   Sagittal T1 fat-saturated Gad+

Case 47

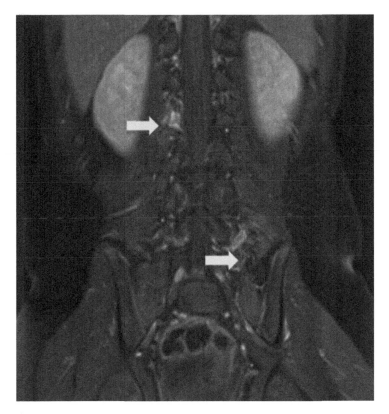

Fig. 47.2 Coronal T1 fat-saturated Gad+

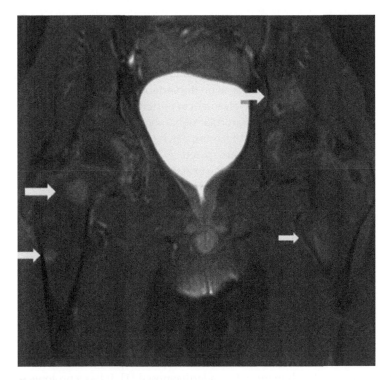

Fig. 47.3 Coronal T1 fat-saturated Gad+

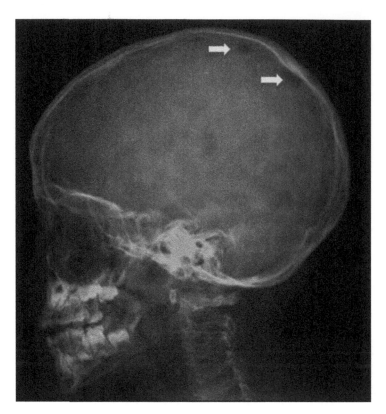

◘ Fig. 47.4 Lateral skull conventional radiograph

Diagnosis Chronic recurrent multifocal osteomyelitis (CRMO)

✔ Answers to Questions

1. Multiple focal lesions with osteolytic behaviour (hypointense on T1-weighted image and with post-contrast enhancement) are seen on the vertebral body of L5 (with partial collapse, involvement of posterior elements, epidural extension and periarticular signal abnormalities), posterior elements of L2, both femurs, pelvic bones and skull. The intervertebral disks are spared.
2. Infectious osteomyelitis (subacute and chronic), Langerhans cell histiocytosis, lymphoproliferative diseases (including leukaemia and lymphoma) and Ewing sarcoma.
3. Complete blood count analysis was normal and blood cultures were negative; there was a slight increase in inflammatory markers. The anatomic pathology diagnosis of the osseous biopsy was consistent with CRMO.

47.1 Comments

CRMO is an idiopathic inflammatory disorder of the bone seen primarily in children and adolescents [1]. True prevalence remains unclear and is thought to be underdiagnosed [1]. It has a prolonged and unpredictable clinical course, with the majority of patients remaining healthy between recurrent episodes [2]. Most patients undergo spontaneous resolution in a number of months to several years. Imaging findings are nonspecific, remaining as an exclusion diagnosis [2]. It presents with multifocal, bilateral and symmetrical osteolytic lesions, predominantly affecting long bones, with different grades of sclerosis and periosteal reaction [2]. Unlike infectious osteomyelitis, it does not typically extend across the intervertebral disk space, with no abscess formation or fistulas [2]. Diagnosis of Langerhans cell histiocytosis (namely, in the form of eosinophilic granuloma) must be considered in this age group, as it remains the principle cause of *vertebra plana*, frequently presenting with associate asymptomatic lytic lesions of skull bones. Biopsy and culture of osseous lesions are required to establish the diagnosis of CRMO and to exclude infectious or malignant infiltration, namely, leukaemia or lymphoma [1].

References

1. Roderick MR, Ramanan AV. Chronic recurrent multifocal osteomyelitis. Adv Exp Med Biol. 2013;764:99–107.
2. Khanna G, Sato TS, Ferguson P. Imaging of chronic recurrent multifocal osteomyelitis. Radiographics. 2009;29(4):1159–77.

Case 48

Daniel Dias

© Springer International Publishing AG 2018
J. Xavier et al. (eds.), *Diagnostic and Therapeutic Neuroradiology*,
https://doi.org/10.1007/978-3-319-61140-2_48

A 16-year-old athlete (volleyball), with chronic low back pain

❓ Questions

1. Identify the affected structure
   A. Pars interarticularis
   B. Inferior articular process
   C. Lamina
   D. Pedicle
2. Which of the following is not associated with this type of lesion?
   A. Sports
   B. Young patient
   C. Spondylolysthesis
   D. Osteoma osteoid
3. What is the diagnosis?
   A. Spondylolysis
   B. Pediculolysis
   C. Laminolysis
   D. Pseudoanterolisthesis

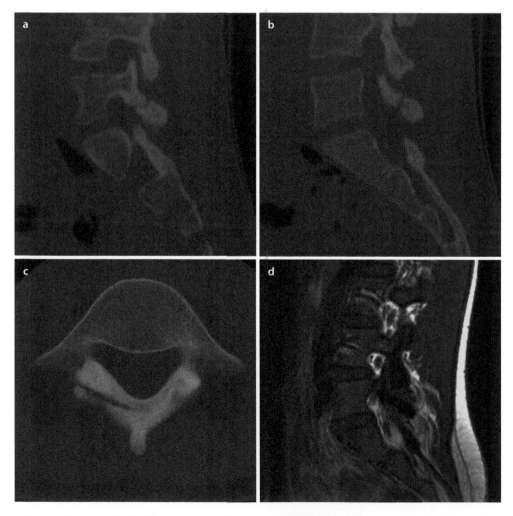

▢ Fig. 48.1 **a** CT scan, sagittal **b** CT scan, sagittal **c** CT scan, axial **d** MRI, sagittal T1

Diagnosis   Laminolysis

 Answers

1. C
2. D
3. C

48.1 Comments

Lumbar stress fractures are a common cause of low back pain in adolescent and young adult athletes. Bony defects can occur at pars interarticularis (spondylolysis), pedicles (pediculolysis) or lamina (laminolysis or retroisthmic cleft). The retroisthmic cleft is a cleft in the lamina immediately dorsal to the inferior processus articularis (❑ Figs. 48.1a, b, c) and is the rarest form of spinal column defect. Although it was formerly considered to be congenital, evidence shows that laminolysis is the result of a preceding stress fracture [1, 2].

There are two types of laminolysis: the hemilaminar type is thought to be subsequent to contralateral spondylolysis, whereas the intralaminar type may be a result of a stress fracture due to repetitive extension loading. The former has a cleft in the unilateral pars, and the latter has a coronal fracture line though both laminae [2].

For correct diagnosis, multidetector three-dimensional computed tomography (CT) is suggested. In addition, magnetic resonance imaging (MRI) also allows detection of inflammation within the defect (❑ Fig. 48.1d).

Patients with spondylolysis are treated conservatively with relative rest, abstinence from sports, and use of a trunk brace. Similar to spondylolysis, conservative treatment is also effective for pain relief in patients with laminolysis [2, 3].

References

1. Wick LF, Kaim A, Bongartz G. Retroisthmic cleft: a stress fracture of the lamina. Skelet Radiol. 2000;29:162–4.
2. Miyagi R, Sairyo K. Two types of laminolysis in adolescent athletes. J Orthop Traumatol. 2012;13(4):225–8.
3. Sakai T, Sairyo K, Takao S, Kosaka H, Yasui N. Adolescents with symptomatic laminolysis: report of two cases. J Orthop Traumatol. 2010;11(3):189–93.

Case 49

João Xavier

References – 266

Below are CT images of a 49-year-old woman's lumbar spine:

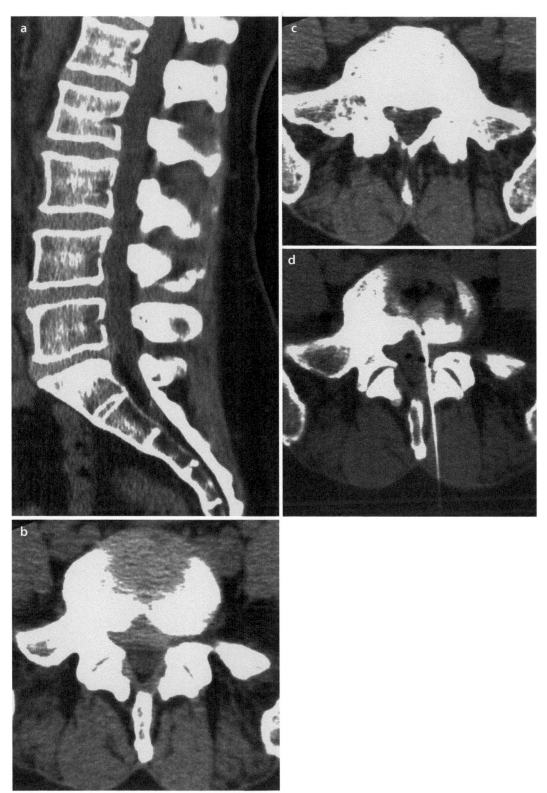

◘ Fig. 49.1   **a** middle line sagittal slice; **b–d** axial slices at L5-S1 level

❓ Question 1: What are the findings?
- (a) Multilevel disc bulging.
- (b) Right subarticular disc herniation at L5-S1.
- (c) Vacuum degenerative disc disease at L5-S1.
- (d) a and b are correct.
- (e) a, b and c are correct.

❓ Question 2: Only based on these images, which of the following could be the patient complains?
- (a) Low back pain.
- (b) Right sciatic pain.
- (c) Left sciatic pain.
- (d) a and b are possible.
- (e) All are possible.

❓ Question 3: Why is a needle inserted in the nucleus pulposus through the epidural space (◘ Fig. 49.1d)?
- (a) Someone tried to do a lumbar puncture, but the target was missed.
- (b) I am not sure if it is a needle. It may be another type of strange body.
- (c) It must be a chemodiskolysis procedure.
- (d) It must be a disc biopsy.
- (e) c and d are correct.

Diagnosis *Multilevel disc degenerative disease* (easy, was it not?)

✅ **Answers and Discussion (and Embedded Captions)**

Question 1: d

Sagittal image (◨ Fig. 49.1a) shows multilevel disc bulging; axial slices (◨ Figs. 49.1b, c) show disc bulging at L5-S1 (maybe a protrusion) and right subarticular disc herniation below disc level. The gas density inside disc (◨ Fig. 49.1d) is iatrogenic (see below).

Question 2: e

Disc disease can produce low back pain due to disc degeneration, annular tears or endplate changes [1]. It is very likely that there is a right S1 root compression (see ◨ Fig. 49.1c), but a left S1 root compression is also possible. Intervertebral foramina (not shown) were also reduced but without evidence of root compression (however, it should be taken into account that the examination position is dorsal decubitus, which has different forces than when standing). This patient had an ill-defined pain in left L5/S1 distribution, which stresses the fact that pain depends on the mechanical compression and on the inflammatory process. If the latter is not present, there will be no pain (besides, the extruded material tends to spontaneously shrink, so, often, one only has to overcome the acute phase). The right subarticular disc herniation had been known for 9 years, when the patient had a right S1 crisis, but she had been asymptomatic since that episode.

Question 3: c

Of course it is a needle! Lumbar punctures are usually performed at L4-L5 level without image guidance, and we are not so incautious as to reach the intervertebral disc when performing them! The needle is a thin one (22G). For biopsy, a larger device is needed (usually 14–20G). This was a chemodiskolysis procedure, by injection of an oxygen-ozone mixture (the gas density seen on ◨ Fig. 49.1d), under CT guidance. Ozone is a cheap and safe material, which has a double effect on disc disease: it shrinks the disc (the disc becomes «mummified») and has a strong anti-inflammatory effect [1, 2]. Disc puncture can be done by a paravertebral or translaminar/transligamentar approach [1]. At L5-S1 level, the safer paravertebral approach is not straightforward because of the ala of the sacrum, but a fine needle can pass through the epidural space and reach the disc, allowing an appropriate injection of the mixture. In this case, the left transligamentar puncture was preferred as the pain was on the left side, recommending a higher mixture diffusion on this side.

References

1. Muto M, editor. Interventional neuroradiology of the spine – clinical features, diagnosis and therapy. Italia: Springer; 2013.
2. Andreula C, Muto M, Leonardi M. Interventional spinal procedures. Eur J Radiol. 2004;50:112–9.

Case 50

Mario Muto and Gianluigi Guarnieri

© Springer International Publishing AG 2018
J. Xavier et al. (eds.), *Diagnostic and Therapeutic Neuroradiology*,
https://doi.org/10.1007/978-3-319-61140-2_50

A 63-year-old woman affected by left cervicobrachialgia with sensory and motor loss in the last 45 days, resistant to medical therapy (◘ Figs. 50.1, 50.2, and 50.3).

? Questions

1. What are the findings on these MR images?
2. What are the findings on these CT images?

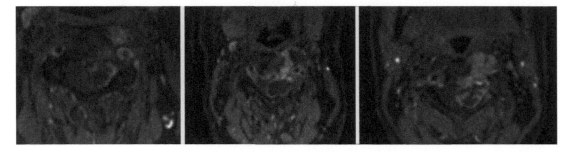

◘ **Fig. 50.1**   axial T1W fat sat-MRI with c.e shows a neoplastic tissue involving C2-C3-C4, anterior and posterior elements

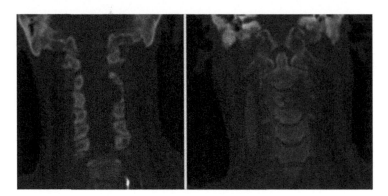

◘ **Fig. 50.2**   coronal and sagittal MPR-MDCT reformat. confirm a huge lytic lesion involving the vertebral body and left elements of C2-C3-C4

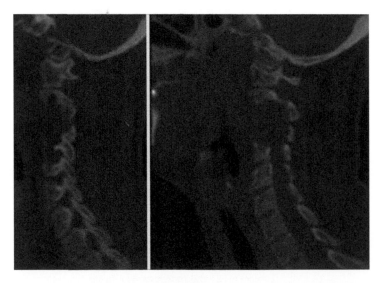

◘ **Fig. 50.3**   coronal and sagittal MPR-MDCT reformat. confirm a huge lytic lesion involving the vertebral body and left elements of C2-C3-C4

Diagnosis   Spinal Chordoma

✅ **Answers**

1. The MRI showed a well-circumscribed lesion involving anterior and posterior spinal elements from C2 to C4 levels on the left side, with low signal intensity on T1W MRI and small foci of hyperintensity (intratumoural haemorrhage or a mucus pool). The axial T1W MRI with contrast agent shows heterogeneous enhancement with a honeycomb appearance corresponding to low T1 signal areas within the tumour. The lesion has mass effect on the spinal cord with contralateral dislocation. The spinal cord has swelling morphology.

2. The MDCT MPR reconstructions show a well-circumscribed destructive lytic lesion involving anterior and posterior spinal elements from C2 to C4 levels on the left side, with moderate enhancement and mass effect on the spinal cord.

50.1 Comments

Chordomas are locally aggressive primary malignant neoplasms that account for 1% of intracranial tumours and 4% of all primary bone tumours [1].

They are midline tumours arising from primitive notochord, the most common site being the sacrum, followed by the clivus and spine (15%). Occasionally they are in an off-midline location.

They are slow growing tumours and present due to mass effect on adjacent structures (brainstem, spinal cord) or as a mass (e.g. sacrococcygeal chordoma).

There are two forms: typical and chondroid.

Pathology: physaliphorous cells containing mucin, calcifications and glycogen vacuoles. Chondroid type has more stromal hyaline content. Both types are positive to epithelial membrane and cytokeratin antigen.

Chordomas of the vertebral bodies are rare, but after lymphoproliferative tumours, they are nonetheless the most common primary malignancy of the spine in adults. They most commonly involve the cervical spine (particularly C2), followed by the lumbar spine then the thoracic spine. They often extend across the intervertebral disc space, involving more than one vertebral segment. They may extend into the epidural space, compressing the spinal cord, or along the nerve roots, enlarging the neural exit foramen [2].

MRI and CT scan have complementary roles in tumour evaluation. CT evaluation is needed to value bone involvement or destruction and to detect patterns of calcification within the lesion. MRI provides excellent 3-dimensional analysis of the posterior fossa (especially the brainstem), sella turcica, cavernous sinuses and middle cranial fossa.

Surgical resection is the first line of treatment in feasible scenarios or a combination of radiation therapy and complete or subtotal surgical resection for selected patients [3, 4].

Prognosis is poor, due to the locally aggressive nature of these tumours, with the 10-year survival being approximately 40%.

References

1. Farsad K, Kattapuram SV, Sacknoff R, et al. Sacral chordoma. Radiographics. 2009;29(5):1525–30.
2. Murphey MD, Andrews CL, Flemming DJ, et al. From the archives of the AFIP. Primary tumors of the spine: radiologic pathologic correlation. Radiographics. 1996;16(5):1131–58.
3. Amendola BE, Amendola MA, Oliver E, et al. Chordoma: role of radiation therapy. Radiology. 1986;158(3):839–43.
4. Fischbein NJ, Kaplan MJ, Holliday RA, et al. Recurrence of clival chordoma along the surgical pathway. AJNR Am J Neuroradiol. 2000;21(3):578–83.

50

Metabolic and Toxic Diseases

Contents

Case 51

Pilar da Cruz and Cristina Ramos

© Springer International Publishing AG 2018
J. Xavier et al. (eds.), *Diagnostic and Therapeutic Neuroradiology*,
https://doi.org/10.1007/978-3-319-61140-2_51

A 46-year-old woman with somnolence, depression and history of liver cirrhosis

❓ Questions

1. What are the relevant findings on these MR images?
2. What is the differential diagnosis?
3. What is the entity in this case and what is the definitive treatment?

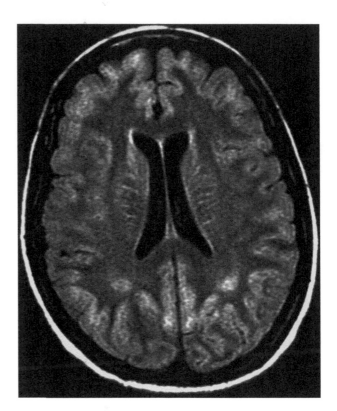

◘ **Fig. 51.1** Axial FLAIR

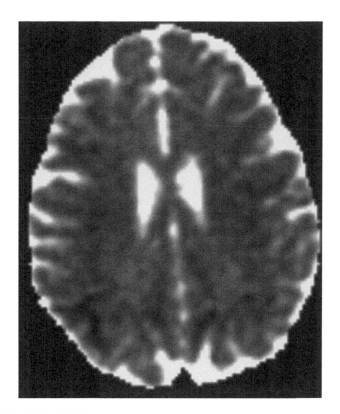

Fig. 51.2 ADC Map

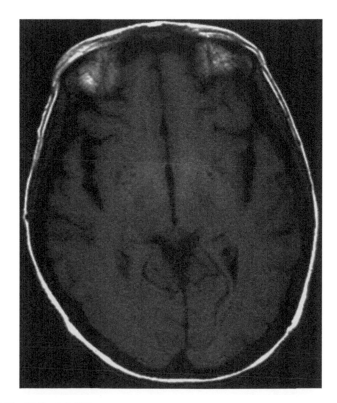

Fig. 51.3 Axial T1

51

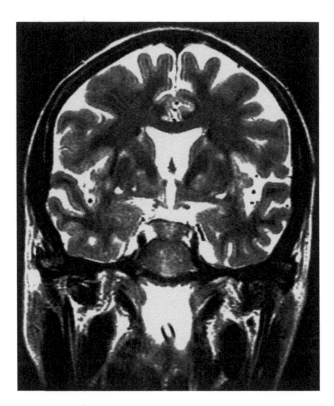

◨ Fig. 51.4   Coronal T2

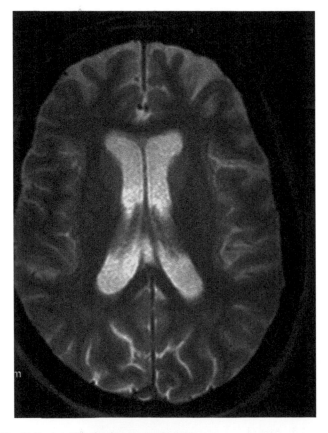

◨ Fig. 51.5   Axial T2 after liver transplantation

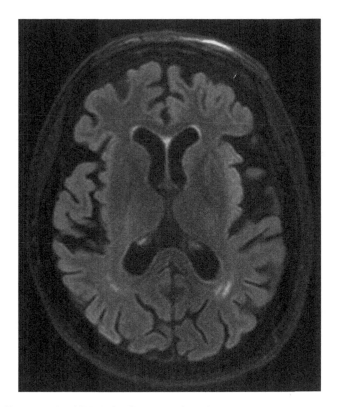

Fig. 51.6 Axial FLAIR after liver transplantation

Diagnosis Hepatic encephalopathy

Answers to Questions

1. Diffuse cortical and subcortical oedema and hyperintensity in FLAIR (Fig. 51.1) with restricted diffusion on ADC map (Fig. 51.2) and T1 and T2 hyperintensity in the basal ganglia (Figs. 51.3 and 51.4).

2. Other toxic and metabolic encephalopathies: disorders of glucose metabolism and disorders of water and electrolyte metabolism; drug overdose and toxic exposures should also be considered.

3. Hepatic encephalopathy; liver transplantation is the definitive treatment.

51.1 Comments

Hepatic encephalopathy (also known as portosystemic encephalopathy) refers to a spectrum of neuropsychiatric abnormalities occurring in patients with liver dysfunction and portal hypertension [2]. It results from exposure of the brain to excessive amounts of ammonia and deposition of manganese. Most patients have a history of chronic cirrhosis with portal hypertension and iatrogenic or spontaneous portosystemic shunts, resulting in nitrogenous waste products crossing the blood-brain barrier and causing long-term toxic brain damage. The basal ganglia may be affected in patients with liver dysfunction.

Characteristic MR imaging signs of acute brain damage may be present in patients with acute hyperammonemia, including cirrhotic patients with acute hepatic decompensation (in whom the ammonia concentration can suddenly increase fourfold) and patients with ornithine transcarbamylase deficiency (i.e. inborn errors of metabolism such as citrullinemia, which result in the accumulation of ammonia in the brain) [1].

Classic MR imaging abnormalities include high signal intensity in the basal ganglia on T1-weighted images (◘ Fig. 51.3), likely a reflection of increased tissue concentrations of manganese.

Acute hyperammonemia causes bilaterally symmetric swelling, T2 prolongation and restricted diffusion in the basal ganglia, insular cortex and cingulate gyrus.

These MR imaging abnormalities probably reflect the presence of mild diffuse brain oedema and may be reversible after liver transplantation (◘ Figs. 51.5 and 51.6).

References

1. Hedge AN, et al. Differential diagnosis for bilateral abnormalities of the basal ganglia and thalamus. Radiographics. 2011;31:5–30.
2. Rovira A, Alonso J, Córdoba J. MR imaging findings in hepatic encephalopathy. Am J Neuroradiol. 2008;29(9):1612–21.

Case 52

Gonçalo Basílio, Lia Neto, and Joana Tavares

© Springer International Publishing AG 2018
J. Xavier et al. (eds.), *Diagnostic and Therapeutic Neuroradiology*,
https://doi.org/10.1007/978-3-319-61140-2_52

A 76-year-old woman with a history of insulin-dependent diabetes mellitus was found at home in an unresponsive state (Glasgow 3). The Boehringer Mannheim (BM) test performed by paramedics at the scene was 30 mg/dL. The patient was immediately administered 40 mL of a 30% glucose infusion and taken to our hospital.

? Questions

1. What is the differential diagnosis?
2. Which areas are typically and specifically spared in this condition?
3. How can the rapid correction of the glucose levels help?

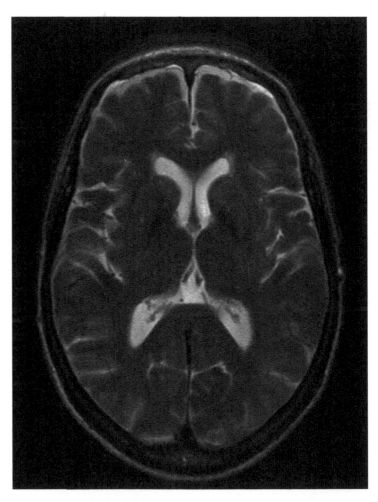

◻ **Fig. 52.1** T2 axial – symmetric hyperintense lesions within the basal ganglia and frontoparietal cortex

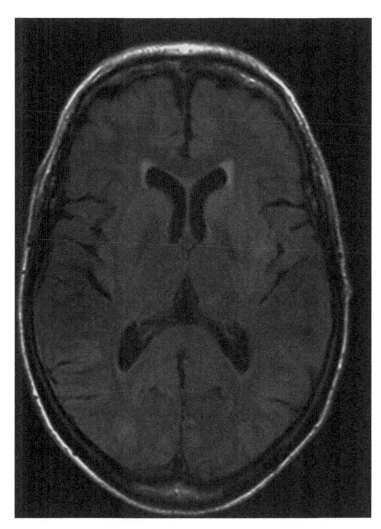

◨ **Fig. 52.2**   FLAIR axial – symmetric hyperintense lesions within the basal ganglia and frontoparietal cortex

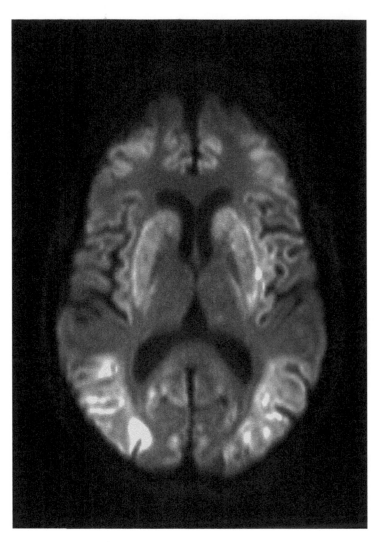

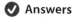 **Fig. 52.3** T2 axial-b1000 axial – restricted diffusion in the same areas of the hyperintensities shown in FLAIR and T2

Diagnosis   Hypoglycaemic encephalopathy

✅ **Answers**
1. Acute cerebral ischaemia, hypoglycaemic encephalopathy and hypoxic-ischaemic brain injury
2. The thalami and the brain stem are usually spared in hypoglycaemic encephalopathy but can be affected in the other differentials (■ Figs. 52.1, 52.2 and 52.3).
3. Rapid diagnosis and early treatment are related to the limitation of neuronal damage.

52.1 Comments

Hypoglycaemic encephalopathy in adult diabetics on insulin is typically due to coma. It is caused by insulin replacement therapy, either through inadequate glucose intake or excessive glucose utilisation (e.g. the accumulation/release of excitatory neurotransmitters increases glucose utilisation). Although less frequent, it can also be due to oral hypoglycaemic medication.

It mainly affects the parietal/occipital lobes (◘ Fig. 52.1, 52.2 and 52.3), hippocampi and amygdala. If severe, it can also affect the globus pallidus and striatum (◘ Fig. 52.1, 52.2 and 52.3). The thalami and the brain stem are usually spared (◘ Fig. 52.1, 52.2 and 52.3).

On MR parietal/occipital gyral swelling with sulci effacement (posterior predominance), [1] can be seen. In acute setting there is restricted diffusion with transient ADC reduction [2] (◘ Fig. 52.3). Later, laminar necrosis may occur with T1 gyral hyperintensity. On MRS NAA may be reduced with high lactate. Usually no haemorrhage is seen.

References

1. Bathla G, Policeni B, Agarwal A. Neuroimaging in patients with abnormal blood glucose levels. AJNR. 2014;35:833–84.
2. Aoki T, Sato T, Hasegawa K, Ishizaki R, Saiki M. Reversible hyperintensity lesion on diffusion-weighted MRI in hypoglycemic coma. Neurology. 2004;63(2):392–3.

Case 53

Carolina Pinheiro, Mariana Cardoso Diogo, and Carla Conceição

© Springer International Publishing AG 2018
J. Xavier et al. (eds.), *Diagnostic and Therapeutic Neuroradiology*,
https://doi.org/10.1007/978-3-319-61140-2_53

A 28-year-old man with a history of alcohol abuse and cannabis use was found unconscious, after drinking home-made wine for three consecutive days and admitted to the emergency room with a Glasgow Coma Scale of 5 and a metabolic acidosis (◘ Figs. 53.1, 53.2 and 53.3).

❓ Questions
1. What are the findings?
2. What is the differential diagnosis of putaminal necrosis?
3. What is the expected prognosis?

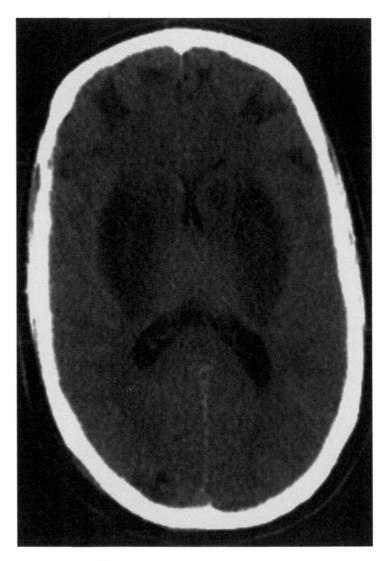

◘ Fig. 53.1   Axial brain-CT scan

53

Case 53

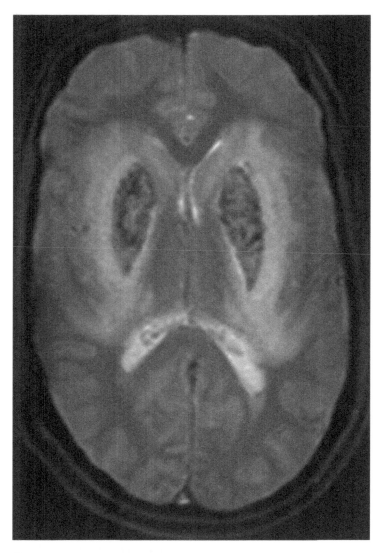

◘ Fig. 53.2   Axial gradient-echo T2*-weighted MRI

53

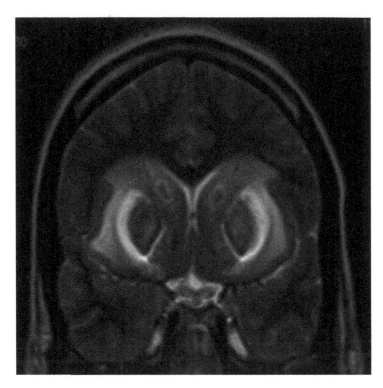

⬛ Fig. 53.3 Coronal T2-weighted MRI

Diagnosis   Methanol intoxication

✓ Answers to the Questions

1. Brain-CT shows bilateral symmetrical hypodensities of the basal ganglia with punctuate putaminal hyperdensities consistent with haemorrhage. It also reveals hypodensity in the subcortical white matter and caudate nuclei. On MRI, T2*WI shows lenticular nuclei necrosis with haemorrhage, and the T2 coronal view shows optic chiasm oedema.

2. Wilson disease, Leigh disease, Kearns-Sayre syndrome, carbon monoxide inhalation, hypoxic-ischaemic injury, acute cyanide intoxication, ADEM, some organic acidopathies and osmotic demyelination osmotic demyelination syndrome.

3. Mortality rate is around 84% in patients with initial presentation of coma and seizure.

53.1 Comments

Methanol is a colourless, highly toxic liquid with a similar smell and taste to ethanol [1]. It is obtained from wood distillation and frequently used as a solvent [2]. Intoxication ensues after accidental or suicidal ingestion of industrial solvents or ingestion of adulterated alcoholic beverages. Symptoms of methanol ingestion include nausea, headache, blurred vision and altered mental status [2]. Anion-gap metabolic acidosis is commonly present. Severe poisoning induces permanent neurological sequelae such as optic neuropathy, leading to blindness, seizure, coma and death [2]. Bilateral putaminal necrosis is a rarely reported, but characteristic, imaging finding [2]. It can be associated with haemorrhage and subcortical white matter lesions, seen only in patients who survive for more than 24 h, and are associated with a poor clinical outcome. Treatment aims at preventing conversion of methanol into toxic metabolites by administrating ethanol [1] or fomepizole [2]. Other therapeutic procedures include gastric lavage, correction of acidosis with sodium bicarbonate, folic acid and haemodialysis [1].

References

1. Blanco M, Casado R, et al. CT and MR imaging findings in methanol intoxication. AJNR Am J Neuroradiol. 2006;27:452–4.
2. Singh A, Samson R, et al. Portrait of a methanol-intoxicated brain. Am J Med. 2011;124(2):125–7.

Case 54

Valentina Ribeiro

© Springer International Publishing AG 2018
J. Xavier et al. (eds.), *Diagnostic and Therapeutic Neuroradiology*,
https://doi.org/10.1007/978-3-319-61140-2_54

A 9-year-old boy with movement disorder predominantly affecting the lower limbs, associated with a cerebellar syndrome, cognitive deterioration and myoclonias

? **Questions**
1. What are the findings?
2. What is the differential diagnosis?
3. What are the diseases in this entity?

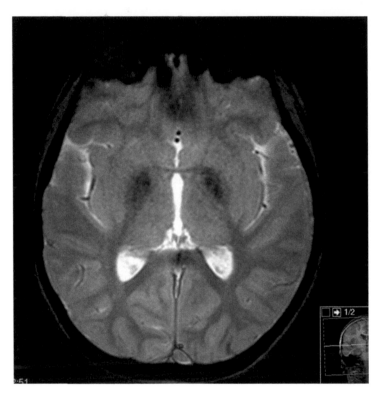

◘ **Fig. 54.1**   Axial T2*

Case 54

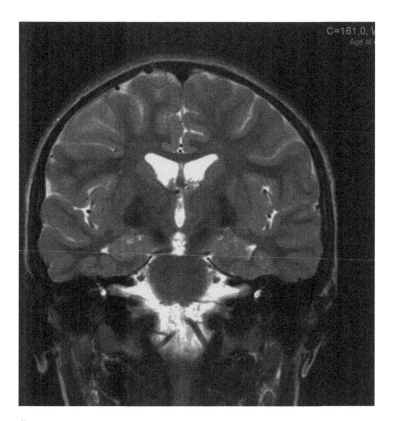

Fig. 54.2 Coronal T2 TSE

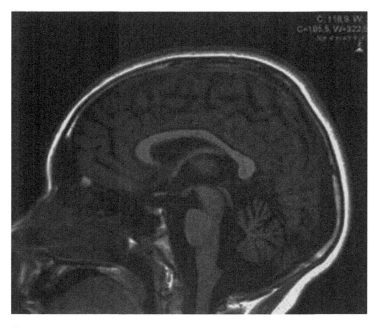

Fig. 54.3 Sagittal T1

Diagnosis Neurodegeneration with brain iron accumulation (NBIA)

✅ **Answers**

1. There is symmetrical hypointensity in the globus pallidi (◪ Fig. 54.1, Axial T2*) and substantia nigra (◪ Fig. 54.2, coronal T2 TSE) compatible with excessive iron deposition and cerebellar atrophy (◪ Fig. 54.3, sagittal T1). Images were obtained on a 3T scanner.

2. Metabolic and degenerative disorders with T2 hypointensity GP: neuronal ceroid lipofuscinosis (cerebellar atrophy) and fucosidosis (white matter atrophy, cutaneous lesions, hepatosplenomegaly). Iron deposition also occurs in multiple sclerosis, human immunodeficiency virus dementia, Friedreich ataxia and Alzheimer and Parkinson diseases.

3. NBIA includes PKAN, PLA2G6-associated neurodegeneration, CoPAN (Coasy protein-associated neurodegeneration), BPAN (beta-propeller-associated neurodegeneration), infantile neuroaxonal dystrophy, aceruloplasminemia, neuroferritinopaty and others (Kufor Rakeb, Woodhouse Sakati, FAHN, SENDA).

54

54.1 **Comments**

NBIA presents with a progressive extrapyramidal syndrome and excessive iron deposition in the brain, particularly affecting the basal ganglia, mainly the globus pallidus. The known causes of NBIA include pantothenate kinase-associated neurodegeneration (PKAN, formerly known as Hallervorden–Spatz disease), neuroferritinopathy, infantile neuroaxonal dystrophy (INAD) and aceruloplasminemia [1].

In this case, a mutation was found in the gene encoding calcium-independent phospholipase A2 (PLA2G6), leading to the diagnosis of INAD. Radiographically, INAD features iron deposition in the globus pallidus and substantia nigra. Significant atrophy of both the cerebellar vermis and hemispheres is a frequent feature and typically precedes iron accumulation.

All patients with PANK2 mutations had the specific pattern of globus pallidus central hyperintensity with surrounding hypointensity on T2-weighted images, known as the eye-of-the-tiger sign [2].

By contrast, neuroferritinopathy has hypointensity involving dentate nuclei, globus pallidus and putamen, with confluent areas of hyperintensity due to probable cavitation, involving the pallida and putamen in 52% of cases, and a subset having lesions in caudate nuclei and thalami [2]. More uniform involvement of all basal ganglia and the thalami is typical in aceruloplasminemia but without cavitation.

MR imaging abnormalities outside the globus pallidus include cerebral or cerebellar atrophy [3].

In the majority of cases, different subtypes of neurodegeneration associated with brain iron accumulation can be reliably distinguished with T2* and T2 fast spin echo brain MRI, leading to accurate clinical and subsequent molecular diagnosis [3].

References

1. Barkovich AJ, Moore KR, Grant E, Jones BV, Vezina G, Koch BL, Raybaud C, Blaser S, Hedlund GL, Illner A. Diagnostic Imaging, Pediatric Neuroradiology. I:1-104–107. Amirsys 2007.
2. Schneider SA, Hardy J, Bhatia KP. Syndromes of neurodegeneration with brain iron accumulation (NBIA): an update on clinical presentations, histological and genetic underpinnings, and treatment considerations. Mov Disord. 2011;27(1):42–53.
3. Hayflick SJ, Hartman M, Coryell J, Gitschier J, Rowley H. Brain MRI in neurodegeneration with brain iron accumulation with and withoud PANK2 mutations. AJNR Am J Neuroradiol. 2006;27:1230–3.

Case 55

Maria Goreti Sá

© Springer International Publishing AG 2018
J. Xavier et al. (eds.), *Diagnostic and Therapeutic Neuroradiology*,
https://doi.org/10.1007/978-3-319-61140-2_55

A 45-year-old woman diagnosed with HCV genotype 3a in 2010, whose condition had worsened in 2013–2014 with hepatocellular insufficiency. In 2015 she suffered acute hepatic failure and encephalopathy grade III, with mild hyponatraemia.

Although there were no surgical complications during the liver transplant, the patient evolved into a comatose state.

❓ Questions
- A. What are the imaging findings?
- B. Which is a main diagnostic hypothesis?
- C. Which laboratorial test would be more useful to support the main diagnostic hypothesis?

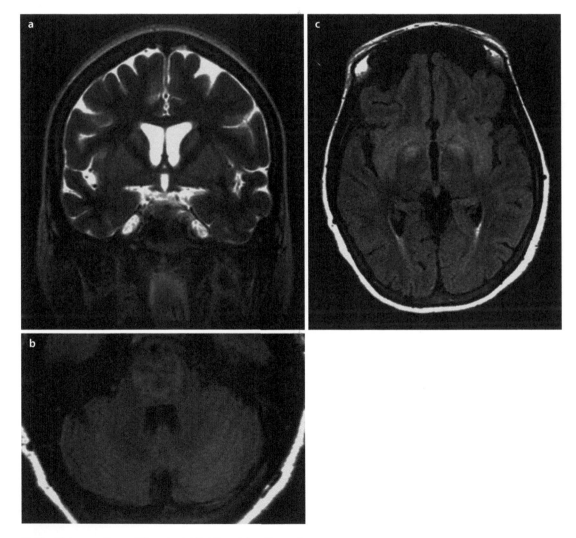

◻ Fig. 55.1   a–c Coronal T2 and axial FLAIR-weighted images

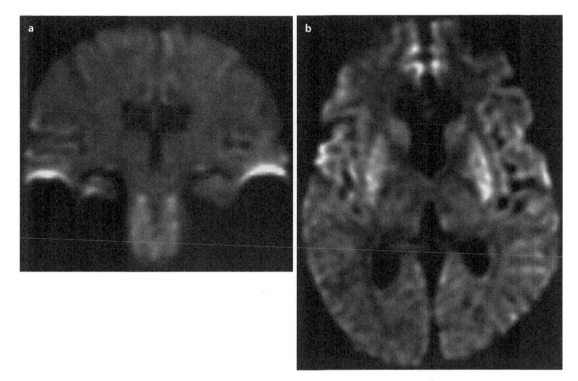

Fig. 55.2 **a, b** Coronal and axial diffusion-weighted images

Diagnosis Osmotic pontine and extrapontine demyelination

✅ Answers

A. The first MRI performed 3 days after liver transplantation showed lesions with high signal intensities in the pons, caudate and lentiform nucleus, thalamus and insular region, in a bilateral and symmetrical pattern. This hyperintensity was demonstrated on T2W (■ Fig. 55.1a), FLAIR (■ Fig. 55.1b, c) and diffusion images (■ Fig. 55.2a, b), with restricted diffusion confirmed in ADC maps. In the lower pons, the hipersinal has a classic trident-shaped appearance (■ Fig. 55.1b).

B. MRI demonstrated symmetrical lesions of central pontine demyelination and extra-pontine myelinolysis (CMP and EMP).
     The MRI appearance of CPM and EPM is so characteristic that it is justified to make the diagnosis on MRI characteristics alone.

C. Blood natremia before and after surgery is essential laboratorial test.

55.1 Comments

The osmotic demyelination syndrome is a complication of the treatment of patients with profound, life-threatening hyponatraemia [1]. The pontine peripheral zhone, as well as periventricular and subpial regions, are spared. It occurs as a consequence of a rapid rise in serum tonicity in individuals with chronic severe hyponatraemia who have made intracellular adaptations to the prevailing hypotonicity. Elevation in serum sodium is the major contributor to the rise in tonicity, but potassium elevation may also contribute [2]. Malnutrition and alcoholism seem to be predisposing factors [1–3].

DWI might have the capability of detecting lesions undetectable on T2, within 24 h, when conventional MRI findings were inconspicuous.

The prognosis is not uniformly bad [2].

References

1. Gocht A, Colmant HJ. Central pontine and extrapontine myelinolysis: a report of 58 cases. Clin Neuropathol. 1987;6:262–70.
2. Brown WD. Osmotic demyelination disorders: central pontine and extrapontine myelinolysis. Curr Opin Neurol. 2000;13(6):691–7.
3. Martin RJ. Central pontine and extrapontine myelinolysis: the osmotic demyelination syndromes. J Neurol Neurosurg Psychiatry. 2004;75:iii22–8.

55

Case 56

Luís Botelho

© Springer International Publishing AG 2018
J. Xavier et al. (eds.), *Diagnostic and Therapeutic Neuroradiology*,
https://doi.org/10.1007/978-3-319-61140-2_56

History   A 28-year-old male with a history of epilepsy and absence seizures starting at the age of 12 presents paroxysms suggesting right focal motor seizures.

❓ Questions

1. What are the abnormal findings on these 3T MR images, and which brain structures are affected?
2. What substances can cause high signal on T1-weighted images? Which one is the most likely source of abnormally high T1 signal in the brain in this case?
3. What are the most probable causes?

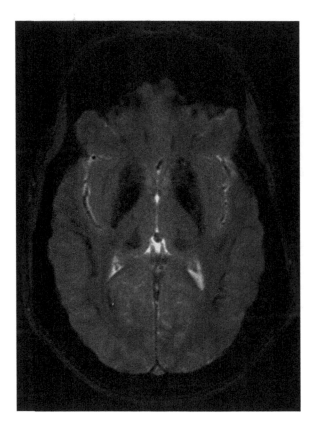

◘ Fig. 56.1   T2-weighted gradient echo

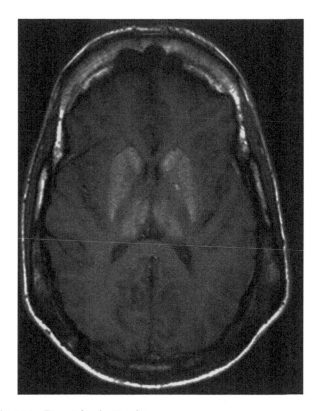

Fig. 56.2 T1-weighted spin echo

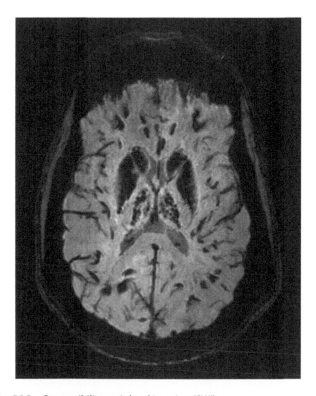

Fig. 56.3 Susceptibility-weighted imaging (SWI)

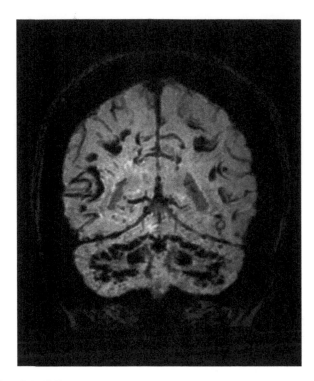

 Fig. 56.4 SWI

Diagnosis Primary hypoparathyroidism

✅ **Answers**

1. The MRI shows extensive abnormal signal changes in the cerebral cortex and cortico-subcortical junction, basal ganglia, thalami, dentate nuclei and subcortical cerebellar white matter. Widespread low signal on T2* (**▣** Fig. 56.1) and SWI (**▣** Figs. 56.3 and 56.4) is seen in these locations. The basal ganglia and thalami reveal increased signal on T1 images. In addition the skull shows enlarged thickness.

2. Common natural causes of T1 shortening and increased signal on T1-weighted images are fat, haemorrhage (methaemoglobin), melanin and neuromelanin, protein-rich content and manganese. Calcium (microcalcification) is also a possible source of T1 shortening and the cause of the higher signal seen in the basal ganglia and thalami in this case (**▣** Fig. 56.2).

3. Disorders of calcium and phosphorous metabolism, hypoparathyroidism, pseudo-hypoparathyroidism, hyperparathyroidism, hypothyroidism, primary familial brain calcification (Fahr disease), mineralising microangiopathy and mitochondrial cytopathies

56.1 Comments

Extensive brain calcifications, as seen in this case, can occur in various processes with different patterns that can overlap. Idiopathic, metabolic, toxic, inherited or infectious diseases are all possible sources of calcification. Idiopathic calcification of the globus pallidus is a common finding seen with advancing age. With more widespread calcification, mitochondrial diseases (MELAS, Leigh disease, Kearns-Sayre syndrome) should be considered, particularly at younger ages. A history of radiotherapy or radiochemotherapy would favour a process of mineralising microangiopathy. An extensive brain involvement, as observed in this case, should prompt the diagnosis of primary familial brain calcification, hypothyroidism, parathyroid and calcium-phosphorus metabolism dysfunction [1, 2].

References

1. Polverosi R, Zambelli C, Sbeghen R. Calcification of the basal nuclei in hypoparathyroidism. The computed and magnetic resonance tomographic aspects. Radiol Med. 1994;87(1–2):12–5.
2. Sobrido MJ, Coppola G, Oliveira J, Hopfer S, Geschwind DH. Primary familial brain calcification. GeneReviews® [Internet]. 2004. [updated 2014 Oct 16] PMID: 20301594.

Case 57

José Eduardo Alves

© Springer International Publishing AG 2018
J. Xavier et al. (eds.), *Diagnostic and Therapeutic Neuroradiology*,
https://doi.org/10.1007/978-3-319-61140-2_57

A 45-year-old female, with a history of severe depression, who lives alone, was absent from work for 2 days in the beginning of October. She resumed work without deficits. One month later, she developed a progressive course of disorientation, behavioral disturbance, and unsteady gait. On neurological examination, the patient showed cognitive deficits (memory, attention, calculus, language) and generalized dystonia.

? Questions

1. What imaging findings most likely explain patient's dystonia?
2. What type of pathological processes causes restricted diffusion in the brain?
3. What two main differential diagnostic groups would you consider in this case?

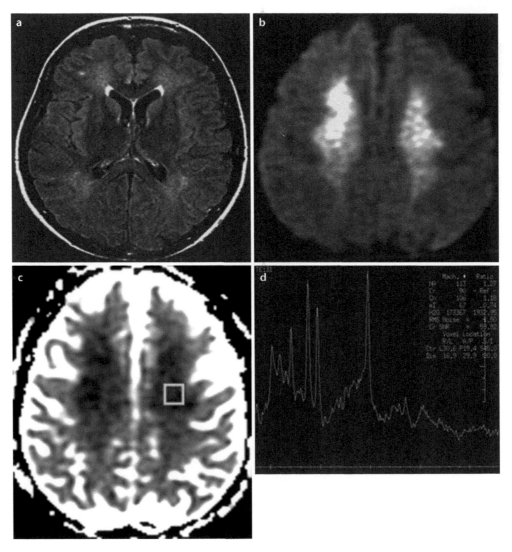

◘ Fig. 57.1   MRI **a** axial T2 FLAIR and **b, c** axial DWI and ADC maps. Short TE single voxel spectroscopy **d**

57

Diagnosis Subacute carbon monoxide poisoning secondary to suicide attempt

Answers

1. Lesions in the striatum.
2. Cytotoxic edema, high cellularity, high viscosity (in fluid collections), intramyelinic edema.
3. Autoimmune and toxic/metabolic disorders.

57.1 Comments

Carbon monoxide poisoning, either intentional or accidental, is one of the most common neurotoxic agents. The pathologic processes related to this entity are complex, including hypoxic-ischemic lesion, inhibition of mitochondrial metabolism, oxidative stress, and lipid peroxidation, responsible for structural alteration of myelin basic protein that culminates in autoimmune demyelination.

This diversity of damaging mechanisms and their occurrence at distinct points of time explain why imaging findings vary over time. In the acute phase, globi pallidi are most commonly affected (atypically, in our patient they were spared), although striatum, thalami, hippocampi, cortex, and even white matter may also be involved (◘ Fig. 57.1a). Lesions present restricted diffusion due to acute ischemia and may show signs of hemorrhagic necrosis (T1 hyper and T2 hypointensity) [1].

In the subacute phase, patients may present with diffuse leukoencephalopathy, affecting mainly centrum semiovale and periventricular white matter, with possible extension to the corpus callosum and subcortical U-fibers. Lesions show restricted diffusion due to ongoing demyelination, have no mass effect, and do not enhance (◘ Fig. 57.1b, c). This subacute leukoencephalopathy explains the delayed neuropsychiatric syndrome (parkinsonism, dystonia, cognitive dysfunction, personality change) which affects 10% of patients exposed to carbon monoxide poisoning after a «lucid interval» of 3–4 weeks (during which there is an apparent full recovery of acute symptoms). MR spectroscopy acquired in the affected white matter consistently shows increased levels of choline, decreased NAA (◘ Fig. 57.1d), and the presence of lactate.

Reference

1. Beppu T. The role of MR imaging in assessment of brain damage from carbon monoxide poisoning: a review of the literature. AJNR. 2014;35:625–31.

Case 58

Pedro Pinto

A 4-year-old girl with normal development until 8 months before when she had an upper respiratory infection with cerebellar ataxia and dyspraxia. On MRI T2-weighted periventricular and subcortical white matter foci were found, and a diagnosis of acute demyelinating encephalomyelitis (ADEM) was proposed. Clinical symptoms totally recovered with corticotherapy. A week ago she started again with mild gait disturbance and came to the emergency department after a minor trauma. Neurological exam showed central cerebellar ataxia, mild paraparesis and visual impairment. MRI was repeated and the images are shown.

❓ Questions

1. What are the main MRI findings?
2. Are cerebellar and supratentorial changes usually similar?
3. What are the main differential diagnoses?

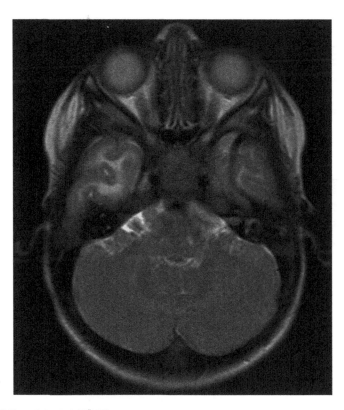

◘ **Fig. 58.1**   Axial T2-WI

Case 58

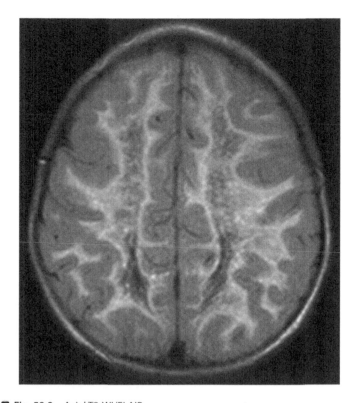

Fig. 58.2 Axial T2-WI/FLAIR

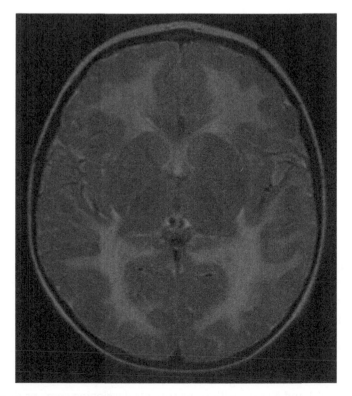

Fig. 58.3 Axial T2-WI

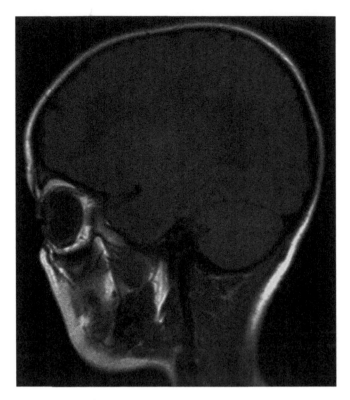

◨ **Fig. 58.4** Sagittal T1-WI

Diagnosis Vanishing white matter disease

✅ **Answers to the questions**

1. Periventricular and subcortical white matter confluent T2-weighted hyperintensity (◨ Figs. 58.1, 58.2 and 58.3) with T1-weighted low central intensity (◨ Fig. 58.4), sparing cortex, basal ganglia and thalami with cystic changes (◨ Fig. 58.2). No cerebral atrophy is found.
2. No. The cerebellum is not always involved and usually does not have cystic changes.
3. ADEM, encephalitis, mitochondrial diseases, metachromatic leukodystrophy, Canavan disease, merosin-deficient congenital muscular dystrophy, Pelizaeus-Merzbacher disease

58.1 Comments

Vanishing white matter is also known as childhood ataxia with CNS hypomyelination disease or myelinopathia centralis diffusa. It is due to mutations in eukaryotic initiation factor 2B (eIF2B). Identification of the genetic defect led to the recognition of a wider clinical spectrum [1]. Early development may initially be normal, new-onset ataxia being the most common symptom between the ages of 1 and 5 years, with some patients developing coma or dysmetric tremor. Subsequently, deterioration is generally progressive with increasing difficulty in walking, spasticity, hyperreflexia, dysarthria and seizures. Optic atrophy develops late in the course of the disease [2]. Typically there is clinically evident sensitivity to febrile infections, minor head trauma and acute fright, which can cause rapid neurological deterioration. Over time, MRI shows evidence of progressive rarefaction and cystic degeneration of the affected white matter, which is replaced by fluid. «Tigroid» pattern is not pathognomonic of this disease but is due to a radiating, stripe-like pattern within the rarefied and cystic white matter, suggesting remaining tissue strands. Contrast enhancement has never been reported. In the end stage of the disease, all cerebral hemispheric white matter may have vanished, leaving the ventricular wall and cortex with intervening fluid. It is striking that even at this end stage, the brain does not collapse and rarely shows evidence of external atrophy. Cerebellar atrophy may occur, but the process of rarefaction and cystic degeneration does not involve the cerebellar white matter and brainstem. There is good correlation between MRI findings and detection of mutations in the EIF2B1-5 genes. There is no specific treatment for this disease. Avoidance of stressful situations known to provoke deterioration is essential, but it is not sufficient to prevent the onset or progression of the disease. Prenatal diagnosis has become available for families as soon as the disease-causing mutations in the index patient are identified.

References

1. van der Knaap MS, Sheper J. Vanishing white matter disease. Lancet Neurol. 2006;5:413–23.
2. Schiffmann R, Elroy-Stein O. Childhood ataxia with CNS hypomyelination/vanishing white matter disease – a common leukodystrophy caused by abnormal control of protein synthesis. Mol Genet Metab. 2006;8:7–15.

Head and Neck

Contents

Case 59

Bruno Moreira

© Springer International Publishing AG 2018
J. Xavier et al. (eds.), *Diagnostic and Therapeutic Neuroradiology*,
https://doi.org/10.1007/978-3-319-61140-2_59

A 51-year-old male with a 2-month history of a right external meatus mild yellowish discharge and suffering,from vertigo in the last week. Physical examination revealed a polypoid lesion filling the external auditory canal (■ Figs. 59.1, 59.2, 59.3 and 59.4).

? Questions

1. Concerning the lesion centred in the right temporal bone, what would be your differentials?
2. Is the vertigo related to this lesion?
3. Should we perform any additional exam to obtain additional clues?

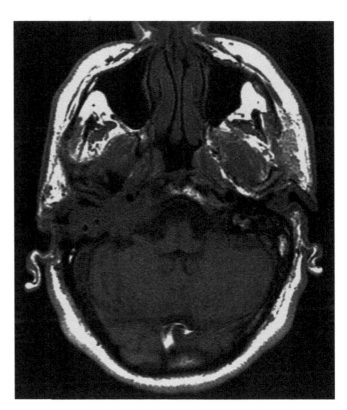

■ Fig. 59.1   Ax T1WI

59

Case 59

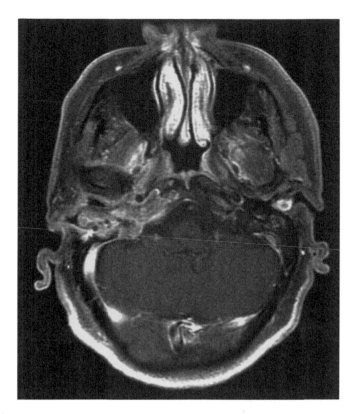

Fig. 59.2 Ax contrast-enhanced T1WI

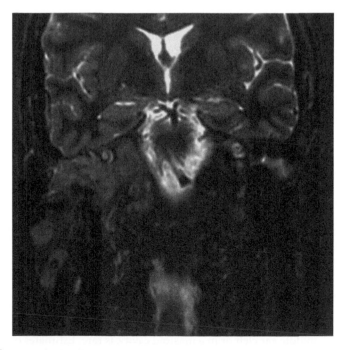

Fig. 59.3 Cor STIRWI

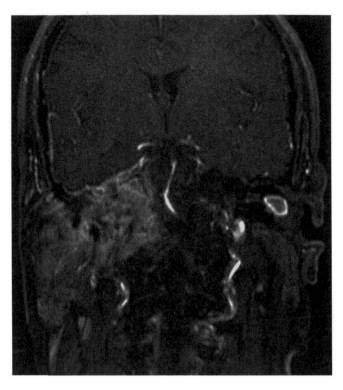

◘ Fig. 59.4   Cor contrast-enhanced T1WI

Diagnosis   Middle ear squamous cell carcinoma

✅ Answers to questions

1. Carcinoma of the middle ear, jugulotympanic paraganglioma, lymphoma, melanoma, nasopharynx/parotid tumour dissemination, metastasis and malignant external otitis.
2. Yes. This lesion partially destroys the basal turn of the cochlea. Therefore, we may have a perilymphatic fistula.
3. If you are concerned about performing a biopsy in a highly vascularized lesion such as a paraganglioma, you should perform a digital subtraction angiography. It shows the intense tumour blush and the feeding vessels, and early draining veins may also be noted due to intra-tumoural shunting. Angiography also has a role to play in preoperative embolization, which is typically carried out 1–2 days prior to surgery.

59.1   Comments

Squamous cell carcinoma of the ear, arising in the external auditory canal, middle ear cleft or in a mastoid cavity, is rare. Estimates of its frequency in the general population vary from 0.004% to 0.0006%, accounting for less than 0.2% of all head and neck malignancies.

59

Nevertheless, squamous cell carcinoma is the most common malignant tumour of the ear. Patients in the fifth to seventh decade are most often affected [2].

Because the middle ear is a cavity within the temporal bone, middle ear carcinoma causes symptoms similar to those of chronic otitis media, making it difficult for clinicians to make an early diagnosis [1].

Primary middle ear carcinoma mainly spreads by direct extension, and distant metastases are rare. Tumours may grow upward through the tegmen tympani into the middle cranial fossa (as in this case, where we find meningeal enhancement in this fossa), anteriorly into the glenoid fossa and infratemporal space, inferiorly into the hypotympanum and jugular foramen, posteriorly to involve the mastoid air cells and medially to involve the carotid canal. Neoplastic cells can also spread along the facial planes of the Eustachian tube and involve the lateral nasopharynx. Interestingly, the erosion of auditory ossicles is not common. The hard avascular bone of the otic capsule is relatively resistant to tumour, and direct invasion of the inner ear signifies far advanced disease (also as in this case) [1].

The therapy of squamous cell carcinoma of the ear and temporal bone depends on the extent of the disease. Middle ear and deeper temporal bone extension are associated with a much poorer prognosis. Subtotal temporal bone resection, possibly in association with radiotherapy, will occasionally result in long-term survival. Local recurrence, followed by intracranial extension, is the most common cause of treatment failure [2].

References

1. Zhang F, et al. Computed tomography and magnetic resonance imaging findings for primary middle-ear carcinoma. J Laryngol Otol. 2013;127(6): 578–83.
2. Friedman DP, et al. MR and CT of squamous cell carcinoma of the middle ear and mastoid complex. AJNR. 1991;12:872–4.

Case 60

Ângelo Carneiro

© Springer International Publishing AG 2018
J. Xavier et al. (eds.), *Diagnostic and Therapeutic Neuroradiology*,
https://doi.org/10.1007/978-3-319-61140-2_60

A 3-year-old child with a bluish mass in his tongue, which first appeared at the age of 4 months and had enlarged ever since

? Questions

1. What are the findings?
2. Which are the most common differential diagnoses?
3. What is the most frequent natural history of this lesion?

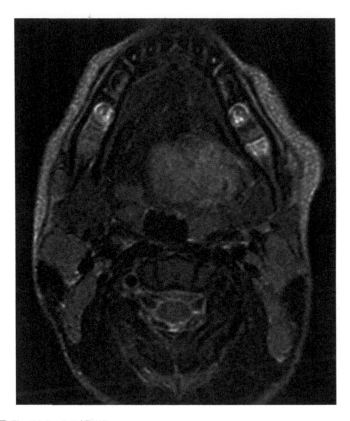

■ **Fig. 60.1** Axial T2WI

Case 60

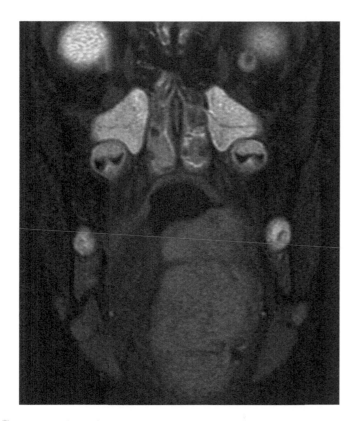

◘ **Fig. 60.2** Coronal STIR

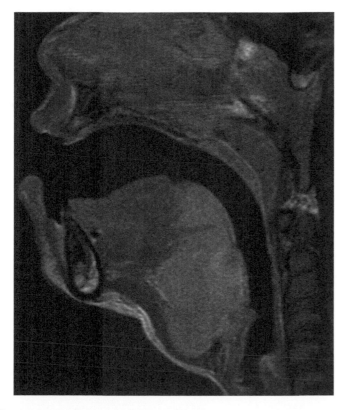

◘ **Fig. 60.3** Sagittal contrast-enhanced T1WI

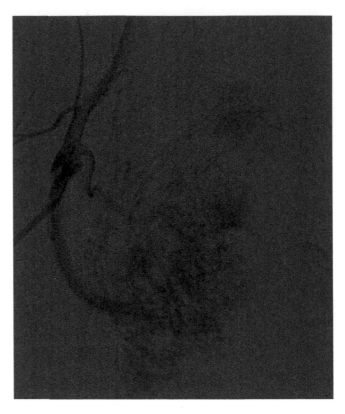

Fig. 60.4   DSA, left external carotid injection, lateral view

60.1   Lingual Infantile Hemangioma

✅ **Answers to Questions**
1. There is a lobulated mass in the posterior third of the tongue, moderately hyperintense on T2WI (■ Figs. 60.1 and 60.2) and well circumscribed. No cysts, fluid-fluid levels, or calcifications can be seen. There are some tiny hypointense dots most likely corresponding to flow voids, due to high vascularization. After contrast (■ Fig. 60.3), there is strong and homogeneous enhancement. Catheter angiography (■ Fig. 60.4) shows a hypertrophied lingual artery and a tumoral blush in the posterior third of the tongue, without early venous filling (i.e., without arteriovenous shunt).
2. Dermoid (typical fat component, with T1WI hyperintensity and chemical shift) and epidermoid cysts (bright lesion on DWI); true vascular malformations (i.e., nonneoplastic, which are typically present at birth, growing along with the patient and which may exhibit phleboliths or cysts)
3. After an initial growth phase, it then enters a plateau. Most lesions regress after the second or third year of age.

60

60.2 Comments

Hemangiomas are true vascular neoplasms, most frequently occurring in the head and neck region.

Typically they are not present at birth and are only detected after the first few months. They initially go through a proliferative phase, with an important and fast growth. In the first or second year, they stop growing, and after that most of them tend to regress, although some may persist or even enlarge [2].

Superficial lesions tend to exhibit a non-pulsating lump with reddish or bluish discoloration. When in deep locations, they can be totally asymptomatic or, depending on the location, may obstruct the airway. Intraosseous lesions can interfere with the normal development of the facial skeleton.

Most lesions can be correctly diagnosed clinically, especially if superficial. Imaging is indicated only in cases of diagnostic uncertainty, deep locations (to assess the relationship with other vital structures), and suspicion of a syndromic association or for treatment planning.

The most frequent imaging findings are lobulated, well-circumscribed mass, moderate T2WI hyperintensity, some flow voids, and avid contrast enhancement.

Since spontaneous involution is the most common scenario, treatment is only recommended for cases of important cosmetic defect, growth impairment, or airway obstruction. Medical management might be achieved with propranolol. Steroids might also be administered topically or injected directly inside the lesion. Other options include sclerotherapy with bleomycin or other sclerosant agents, laser therapy, and surgical excision [1].

References

1. Marler JJ, Mulliken JB. Current management of haemangiomas and vascular malformations. Clin Plast Surg. 2005;32(1):99–116.
2. Behr GG, Johnson C. Vascular anomalies: hemangiomas and beyond—part 1, fast-flow lesions. Am J Roentgenol. 2013;200(2):414–22.

Case 61

Sofia Pina

© Springer International Publishing AG 2018
J. Xavier et al. (eds.), *Diagnostic and Therapeutic Neuroradiology*,
https://doi.org/10.1007/978-3-319-61140-2_61

A 56-year-old woman with renal lithiasis since the age of 21, low bone mineral density, elevated PTH, slightly elevated calcium and phosphorus (◘ Figs. 61.1, 61.2, 61.3, and 61.4)

? Questions

1. Describe the imaging protocol and relevant findings.
2. What is the main goal of imaging studies in hyperparathyroidism?
3. What are the main advantages of CT?

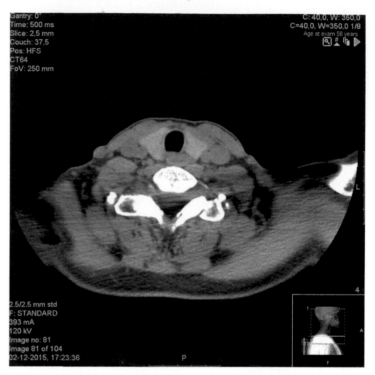

◘ Fig. 61.1   4D-MDCT without contrast

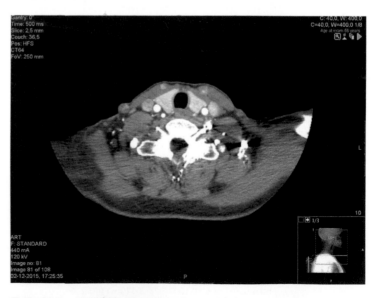

◘ Fig. 61.2   4D-MDCT with contrast, in arterial phase

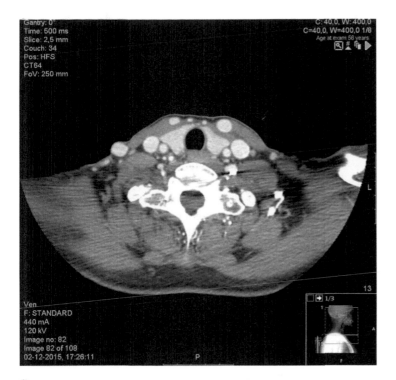

Fig. 61.3 4D-MDCT with contrast, in venous phase

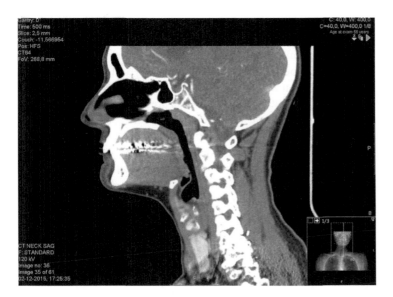

Fig. 61.4 4D-MDCT with contrast, sagital slice in venous phase

Diagnosis Parathyroid adenoma

✅ **Answers**

1. This is a multiphase acquisition technique, introducing
   the time factor to the three-dimensional study; it is called
   4D-MDCT. In recent literature, some studies have shown
   that 4D-MDCT as a dynamic volumetric study is more

effective than sonography and scintigraphy sestamibi, determining the location and lateralisation of parathyroid hyperactive tissue. The findings are an ovoid lesion posterior to the superior left thyroid lobe of approximately 1, 5 cm of cranio-cephalic extension showing rapid wash-in and rapid washout of contrast, typically seen in parathyroid hyperplasia or adenoma.

2. Preoperative localisation and lateralisation of abnormal parathyroid tissue/lesion for identifying patients who are candidates for minimally invasive surgery is the main concern in today's practice.

3. Advantages of 4D-MDCT: Obtaining functional information by contrast enhancement pattern and anatomic detail, taking into account the fact that parathyroid adenomas are distinguishable from other structures of the neck by hyperperfusion or hypervascularisation thereof. High spatial resolution by CT thin slices and volumetric acquisition. Multiplanar reconstruction and 3D allows more precise characterisation of the regional anatomy, planning and access at surgery.

61.1 Comments

Primary hyperparathyroidism is characterised by elevated parathyroid hormone synthesis and release (PTH), resulting in hypercalcemia. Asymptomatic patients are often detected by screening laboratory examinations. The main cause of primary hyperparathyroidism is benign and is due to parathyroid hyperplasia and adenomas. About 80–90% of cases are due to single hyperfunctioning adenoma. Parathyroid carcinomas are rare, occurring in about 1–3% of cases. Multiple lesions occur in 10–14%, and ectopic parathyroid glands occur in 20–25% of cases [1, 2, 3].

Bilateral cervical surgery was the localising procedure initially used and is still being performed today for multiglandular disease (as in MEN1 syndrome). However, the main cause of primary hyperparathyroidism is the single adenoma, and directed parathyroidectomy is progressively being implemented by the availability of preoperative radiological studies with high sensitivity for localisation of the lesion. The imaging study usually performed in patients with primary hyperparathyroidism includes ultrasound and scintigraphy with 99mTc sestamibi (in two phases or using two radiopharmaceuticals). When these studies are negative, CT and magnetic resonance imaging (MRI) of the neck are used in addition to the preoperative investigation. Thus, the CT is used mostly in investigation of ectopic parathyroid glands [1, 2, 3].

The sensitivity of conventional CT is reported in the literature as ranging between 46% and 87%. However, the sensitivity of the 4D-MDCT in detection of abnormal parathyroid glands is 90% [2].

For initial minimally invasive surgery, the preferred localising imaging studies include sestamibi scintigraphy (MIBI-SPECT imaging), ultrasound and/or 4D-MDCT [1, 2, 3].

For all patients undergoing reoperation, it is recommended that preoperative localisation be performed and at least two imaging studies should be obtained to assure concordance under these circumstances [1, 2, 3].

References

1. Greenspan BS, Dillehay G, Intenzo C, Lavely WC, O'Doherty M, Palestro CJ, et al. SNM practice guideline for parathyroid scintigraphy 4.0. J Nucl Med Technol. 2012;40(2):111–8. Epub 2012 Mar 27.
2. Kunstman JW, Kirsch JD, Mahajan A, Udelsman R. Clinical review: parathyroid localization and implications for clinical management. J Clin Endocrinol Metab. 2013;98(3):902–12. https://doi.org/10.1210/jc.2012-3168. Epub 2013 Jan 23.
3. Gafton AR, Glastonbury CM, Eastwood JD, Hoang JK. Parathyroid lesions: characterization with dual-phase arterial and venous enhanced CT of the neck. AJNR Am J Neuroradiol. 2012;33(5):949–52. https://doi.org/10.3174/ajnr.A2885. Epub 2012 Jan 12.

Case 62

José Pedro Rocha Pereira

© Springer International Publishing AG 2018
J. Xavier et al. (eds.), *Diagnostic and Therapeutic Neuroradiology*,
https://doi.org/10.1007/978-3-319-61140-2_62

A 35-year-old female. Otoscopy revealed a reddish pulsatile mass in the middle ear.

❓ Questions

1. What are the main differential diagnoses of a reddish pulsatile mass in the middle ear?
2. What are the image findings?

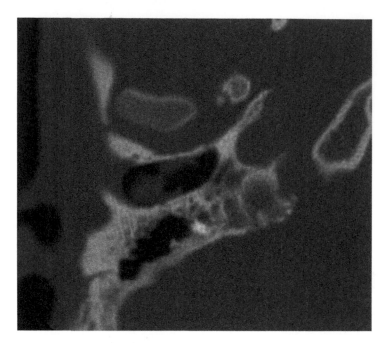

◘ Fig. 62.1   Axial CT carotid canal level

62

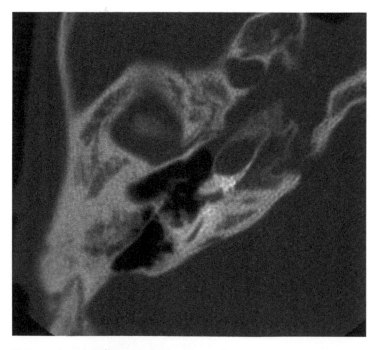

◘ Fig. 62.2   Axial CT hypo-/mesotympanum level

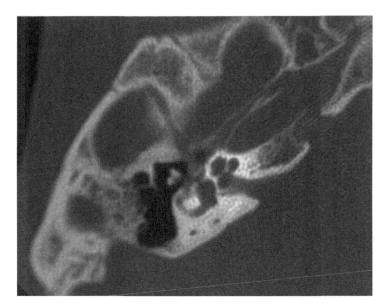

Fig. 62.3   Axial CT epitympanum level

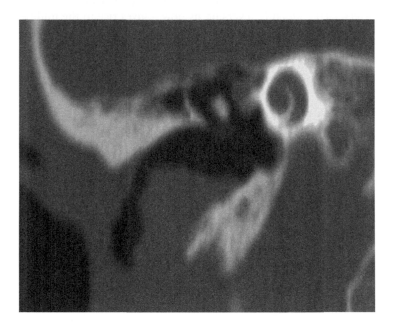

Fig. 62.4   Coronal CT

Diagnosis   Persistent stapedial artery

✓ **Answers**

1. Persistent stapedial artery; paraganglioma; aberrant carotid artery; haemangioma.
2. The images show a «soft tissue» tubular structure with an osseous canal in the petrous segment of the temporal bone (■ Fig. 62.1) that enters the middle ear travelling superiorly along the medial wall (partially inside an osseous canal in the hypotympanum) (■ Fig. 62.2). In the epitympanum, the structure enters the anterior tympanic segment of the facial

nerve (■ Figs. 62.3 and 62.4) and immediately leaves, reaching the middle cranial fossa, where it continues within a sulcus in the squamous part of temporal bone (■ Fig. 62.3). The foramen spinosum is absent. The soft tissue in the external auditory canal is irrelevant.

62.1 Comments

The stapedial artery is an embryonic branch of the petrous segment of the internal carotid artery that reaches the middle cranial base after a short route through the middle ear. Within the middle ear, it passes into the hypotympanum within an osseous canal and then passes through the obturator foramen of the stapes to enter the anterior part of the tympanic segment of the facial canal. After leaving the facial nerve canal, it enters the middle cranial fossa, where it sends out two branches: the maxillomandibular and the supraorbital arteries [2].

The maxillomandibular artery leaves the cranial vault through the foramen spinosum and after joining the future external carotid artery – consequently reversing its flow – gives rise to the middle meningeal artery [2].

The supraorbital artery branches into the marginal artery of the tentorium (which turns posteriorly) and the orbital artery which continues onto the orbit. Either before (in 30% of cases) or after entering the orbit, it divides into the lacrimal and the medial ethmoidonasal arteries. During a later stage of development, the primitive ophthalmic artery takes over these orbital branches of the stapedial system. The transsphenoidal part of the orbital artery partially regresses, and its remnant constitutes a permanent anastomosis between the intraorbital ophthalmic system and the middle meningeal artery [2].

The persistence of the stapedial artery is a rare anatomic variant with unknown prevalence. Its recognition is important to exclude important pathology (such as paraganglioma) and to avoid unnecessary and potentially dangerous surgery [1]. The diagnosis can be made with CT or angiography. The absence of the foramen spinosum may be a good clue for diagnosis, but it can be misleading as it may also be absent when the middle meningeal artery has its origin in the ophthalmic artery.

References

1. Silbergleit R, Quint DJ, Mehta BA, Patel SC, Metes JJ, Noujaim SE. The persistent Stapedial artery. AJNR Am J Neuroradiol. 2000;21:572–7.
2. Lasjaunias P, Berenstein A. Surgical neuroangiography. Vol 1. The skull base and extradural arteries. Berlin: Springer; 1987. p. 414–58.

Case 63

Cláudia Pereira

© Springer International Publishing AG 2018
J. Xavier et al. (eds.), *Diagnostic and Therapeutic Neuroradiology*,
https://doi.org/10.1007/978-3-319-61140-2_63

A 74-year-old diabetic man, complaining of otalgia, dysphagia, and progressive hoarseness

❓ Questions

1. Where is the pathology centered?
2. What is the most likely diagnosis?
3. What is the most helpful imaging feature for the differential diagnosis?
4. Which condition is the most likely cause of this pathology?

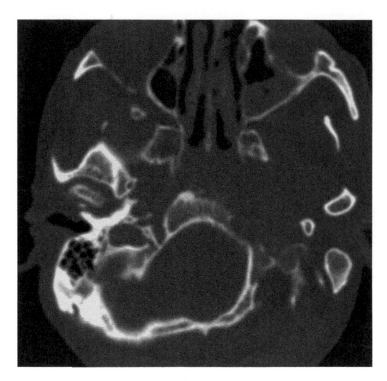

◘ **Fig. 63.1**   Non-contrast head CT, bone window

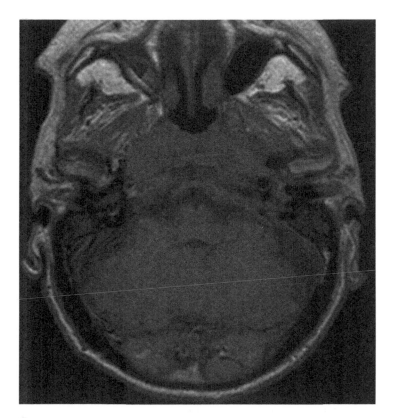

■ Fig. 63.2 T1 axial, without contrast

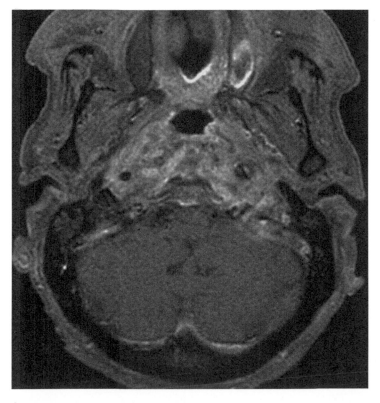

■ Fig. 63.3 Post-contrast axial T1, fat sat

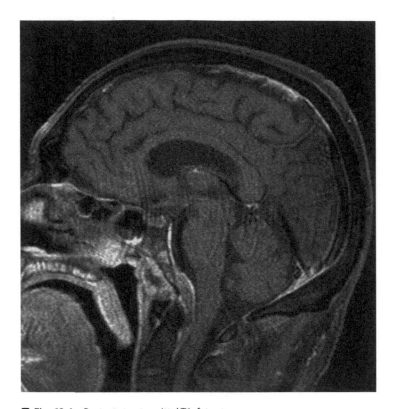

Fig. 63.4 Post-contrast sagittal T1, fat sat

Diagnosis   Skull-base osteomyelitis

✅ **Answers**
1. This pathology is centered at the skull base, mainly at the clivus (◻ Fig. 63.1).
2. Skull-base osteomyelitis.
3. Diffuse clival hypointensity on T1-weighted MR images (◻ Fig. 63.2) and intense contrast enhancement (◻ Figs. 63.3 and 63.4), due to bone marrow infiltration, are characteristic imaging findings.
4. Malignant otitis externa secondary to *Pseudomonas aeruginosa* infection is the most frequent cause of skull-base osteomyelitis.

63.1 Comments

First described in 1959 by Meltzer and Kelemen, skull-base osteomyelitis is an uncommon condition associated with significant morbidity and mortality, which is usually a complication of uncontrolled otogenic, odontogenic, or sinus infection [3].

Patients with this condition usually have underlying conditions which predispose them to infection, such as diabetes mellitus,

corticosteroid use, HIV infection, or chronic inflammatory sphenoid sinus disease. Male patients are most at risk [1].

Headache, otalgia, and cranial neuropathy (as a result of skull-
base foramen involvement) are the most frequent symptoms, while
classic signs of infection (fever, elevated WBC count, positive blood
cultures) are usually absent.

The most consistent MR finding is regional or diffuse clival
hypointensity on T1-weighted images relative to normal fatty marrow and T2 hyperintensity. Although these are not specific, usually
there are also signs of pre- and paraclival soft tissue infiltration,
with obliteration of normal fat planes or even frank soft tissue
masses. Abnormal soft tissue in the cavernous sinus, internal
carotid artery narrowing, meningeal enhancement, as well as signal
intensity abnormality in the adjacent brain parenchyma may also
occur.

Processes to be considered in the differential diagnosis of skull-
base osteomyelitis include squamous cell carcinoma of the head
and neck, lymphoma, hematogenous metastasis, inflammatory
pseudotumor, and granulomatous diseases [2].

A tissue sampling procedure is often required for the definitive
diagnosis of this condition.

References

1. Cheng PC, Fischbein NJ, Holliday RA. Central skull base osteomyelitis in
   patients without otitis externa; imaging findings. AJNR Am J Neuroradiol.
   2003;24:1310–6.
2. Clark MPA, Pretorius PM, Byren I, Milford CA. Central or atypical skull base
   osteomyelitis: diagnosis and treatment. Skull base. 2009;19(4):247–54.
3. Blyth CC, Gomes L, Sorrel TC, Da Cruz M, Sud A, Chen SC-A. Skull-base
   osteomyelitis: fungal vs. bacterial infection. Clin Microbiol Infect.
   2011;17:306–11.

Case 64

Cristiana Vasconcelos

© Springer International Publishing AG 2018
J. Xavier et al. (eds.), *Diagnostic and Therapeutic Neuroradiology*,
https://doi.org/10.1007/978-3-319-61140-2_64

A 53-year-old female with bilateral conductive hearing loss and tinnitus

? Questions
What are the findings?
What is the differential diagnosis?
What is the treatment?

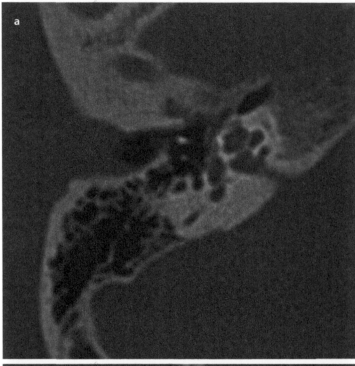

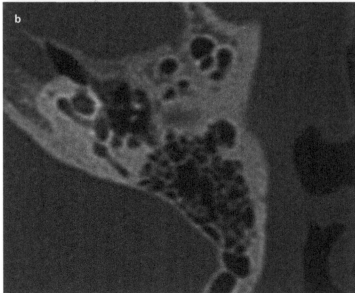

◘ **Fig. 64.1**   Axial computed tomographic images in bone window showing right **a** and left **b** temporal bones

Diagnosis   Fenestral and cochlear otosclerosis

✔ **Answers to Questions**
   1. Bilateral hypodense demineralized plaques are noted in fissula ante fenestram and around the cochlea (◘ Figs. 64.1a, b).
   2. Fenestral otosclerosis has limited differential diagnosis: cochlear cleft (normal variant seen in children) and tympanosclerosis (with post-inflammatory fixation of the stapes). Osteogenesis imperfecta, Paget disease, and otosyphilis rarely mimic cochlear otosclerosis.
   3. Stapedectomy and prosthesis insertion are used to treat fenestral otosclerosis. Fluorides and cochlear implantation are used to treat cochlear otosclerosis.

64.1   Comments

Otosclerosis is also called otospongiosis because the normal ivory-like endochondral bone of the otic capsule is replaced by foci of spongy vascular irregular new bone. These decalcified foci tend to recalcify and become less vascular and more solid. The disease may be inherited by autosomal dominant transmission; however it more commonly occurs as an isolated event, and an inflammatory response likely plays a role in pathogenesis. It is bilateral in approximately 85% of patients. There is a 2:1 female predominance, and it is uncommon among black and oriental people. Patients present in the second to fourth decades of life with conductive hearing loss, sensorineural hearing loss, or mixed hearing loss and/or tinnitus. CT is clearly the mainstay of imaging for otosclerosis, but MRI with contrast shows active osteolysis with enhancement, especially in cochlear otosclerosis, permitting the gauge of activity [1, 2].

The most common lesion in otosclerosis occurs in the region of the fissula ante fenestram, which represents an area of embryonic cartilage that extends from the anterior oval window region to the vicinity of the cochleariform process. The promontory, round window niche, and tympanic segment of the facial nerve may also be involved. The involvement of the annular ligament leads to fixation of the stapes, which is responsible for the typical conductive hearing loss. In 2% of cases, complete obliteration of the oval window may occur. Apart from the size and location of plaques and narrowing of the oval window, the exam report must also include an evaluation of the status of the round window, facial nerve canal, jugular bulb, middle ear cavity, ossicular chain, and inner ear.

Cochlear otosclerosis is a continuum of the fenestral otosclerosis process. Foci of demineralized spongy vascular bone appear in the cochlear capsule and may extend around the vestibule, semicircular canals, and internal auditory canal. It manifests with progressive sensorineural hearing loss.

Complications after stapes surgery include complete displacement of the prosthesis, prosthesis displacement into the vestibule, perilymphatic fistula, and development of reparative granulomas and labyrinthitis. Ossification of the basal turn of the cochlea may be a contraindication for cochlear implant.

References

1. Swartz JD, Loevner LA. Imaging of temporal bone. 4th ed. New York: Thieme; 2009. p. 382–91.
2. Purohit B, Hermans R, Op de Beeck K. Imaging in otosclerosis: a pictorial review. Insights Imaging. 2014;5:245–52.

Case 65

Luís Cardoso, José Eduardo Alves, and Daniel Dias

© Springer International Publishing AG 2018
J. Xavier et al. (eds.), *Diagnostic and Therapeutic Neuroradiology*,
https://doi.org/10.1007/978-3-319-61140-2_65

A 19-month-old female with past history of caesarean birth and congenital ophthalmoparesis noted at 2 months old, with limitation of abduction and vertical gaze of the left eye.

? Questions

1. What are the findings on these MR images?
2. Which clinical hallmarks may be associated with this entity?
3. What is the spectrum of this malformation and can it be graded?

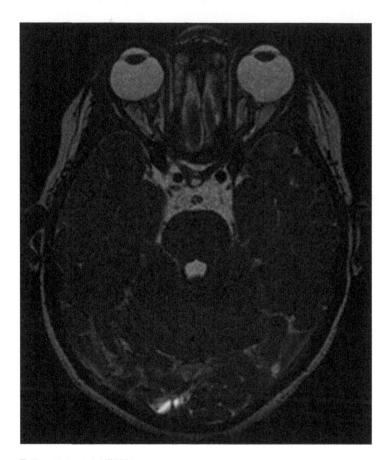

◘ Fig. 65.1   Axial FIESTA

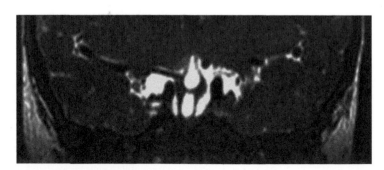

◘ Fig. 65.2   Coronal FIESTA

Case 65

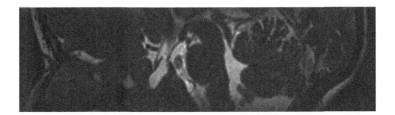

Fig. 65.3 Sagittal FIESTA

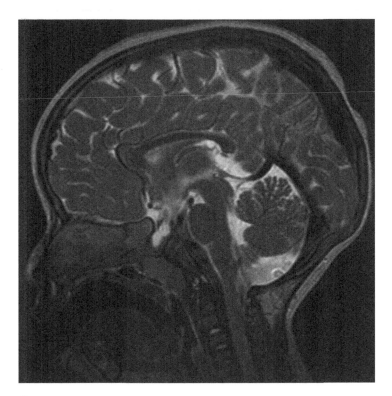

Fig. 65.4 Sagittal T2

Diagnosis Craniopharyngeal canal

✅ Answers to Questions

1. Axial, coronal, and sagittal FIESTA (■ Figs. 65.1, 65.2, and 65.3) and sagittal T2 (■ Fig. 65.4) MR images show a large defect in the midline of the sphenoid bone, with depression of the sella turcica, and a possible communication with the superior wall of the nasopharynx, secondary to bone disruption. The optic chiasm and the infundibular recess of the third ventricle are inferiorly deviated.
2. It might present with associated pituitary dysfunction and secondary hormone abnormalities such as hypopituitarism, growth hormone deficiency, or diabetes insipidus. Congenital midline malformations have also been described.

3. It has been proposed to divide the malformation into three types in order to describe size and pathologic features: small incidental canals (type 1), medium-sized canals containing ectopic adenohypophysis (type 2), large canals with associated cephaloceles (type 3A), tumours of the adeno-hypophysis and associated embryonic tissues (type 3B), or both of these (type 3C).

65.1 Comments

Craniopharyngeal canal is a rare entity characterised by the presence of a tract from the nasopharynx to the pituitary fossa through a well-corticated defect of the midline sphenoid body. It is believed to arise from an error in the normal development of the pituitary gland in which there is a missing obliteration of the adenohypophyseal stalk in continuum with the Rathke's pouch, the precursor of the adenohypophysis, due to an incomplete fusion of the postsphenoid cartilages [1, 2].

Type 1 canals are usually incidental, small, benign findings in patients with other craniofacial or neural congenital anomalies. Type 2 medium-sized and type 3A large canals with cephaloceles are associated with ectopic adenohypophysis and possible pituitary dysfunction. Type 3B canals containing tumours and type 3C containing both tumours and cephaloceles often contain ectopic pituitary tissue within the nasopharynx which should be taken into account during surgery in order to avoid iatrogenic hypopituitarism or CSF leakage. When the clinical assessment shows a nasopharyngeal mass, it may suggest a type 3 canal [1].

References

1. Abele TA, Salzman KL, Harnsberger HR, et al. Craniopharyngeal canal and its spectrum of pathology. AJNR Am J Neuroradiol. 2014;35:772–7.
2. Mehemed TM, Fushimi Y, Okada T, et al. MR imaging of the pituitary gland and postsphenoid ossification in fetal specimens. AJNR Am J Neuroradiol. 2016;37:1523–7.

Miscellaneous (To Find Out for Yourself...)

Contents

Case 66

Marcos Gil da Veiga, Mariana Cardoso Diogo, and Carolina Pinheiro

© Springer International Publishing AG 2018
J. Xavier et al. (eds.), *Diagnostic and Therapeutic Neuroradiology*,
https://doi.org/10.1007/978-3-319-61140-2_66

A 28-year-old woman with β-thalassemia major presented with amenorrhea. She was dependent on regular blood transfusions and deferasirox and deferoxamine administration. At the onset of hypopituitarism, the relevant laboratory results were the following: anaemia (haemoglobin 10.9 g/dL), serum iron 75 mg/mL (60–180), ferritin 8866 ng/mL (11–307), normal TSH, low LH 0,65, and low FSH 1,29. Magnetic resonance (MR) imaging and computerized tomography (CT) of the brain and pituitary gland were performed.

❓ Questions

1. What are the findings?
2. What is the differential diagnosis?
3. Is there an association with other pathologies?

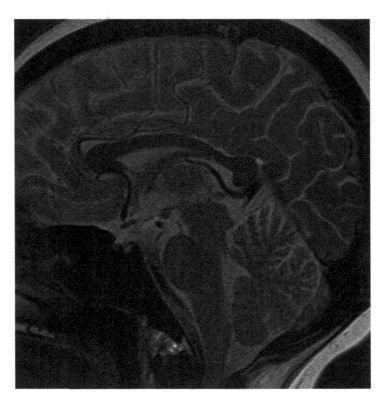

◻ **Fig. 66.1**   Sagittal T2-WI

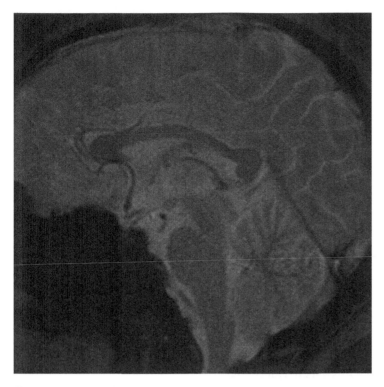

◘ **Fig. 66.2**   Sagittal T2*

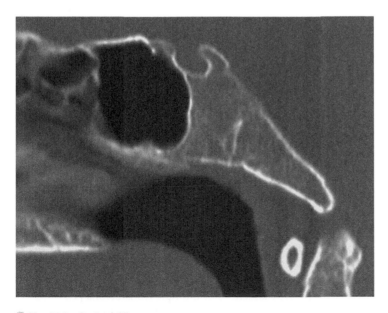

◘ **Fig. 66.3**   Sagittal CT

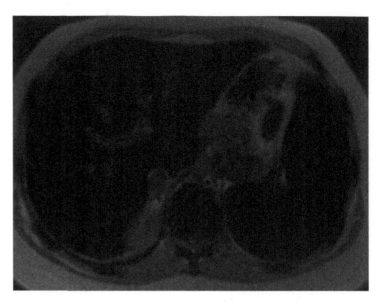

■ **Fig. 66.4** Abdominal Axial T2-WI. Iron quantification was made

Diagnosis   Major β-thalassemia-related hemochromatosis

✅ **Answers to Questions**
1. T2 hypointensity with blooming effect on T2* of the adenohypophysis, superior pineal gland, and skull base (■ Figs. 66.1 and 66.2). Hypointense hepatosplenomegaly, consistent with severe systemic iron overload (■ Fig. 66.3). Iron quantification revealed an iron hepatic concentration of 340 (±50) mol/g.
2. Other entities associated with T2 shortening of the pituitary gland are the following: Hypophysis microadenoma ou macroadenoma, melanoma metastasis, Rathke's cleft cyst, aneurysm, calcification, and craniopharyngioma.
3. Other haematological disorders (haemolytic anaemias, acquired myelodysplastic syndrome) are causes of iron overload that could result in similar imagiological findings.

66.1   Comments

Haemochromatosis is a progressive increase in total body iron with abnormal deposition in multiple organs (■ Fig. 66.3) [1]. Primary haemochromatosis is a rare genetic disorder, whereas secondary haemochromatosis can result from a variety of disorders, such as chronic haemolytic anaemias or multiple transfusions [1].

Thalassaemic syndromes represent the most common causes of ineffective erythropoiesis and secondary iron overload [2]. Additionally, these patients eventually become transfusion dependent [2].

The anterior lobe of the pituitary gland is sensitive to the toxic effects from iron overload, thus resulting in hypopituitarism [2].

Iron deposits cause local magnetic field inhomogeneities with decreased T2 relaxation time and appear hypointense on T2/T2*WI (◨ Figs. 66.1 and 66.2) [1]. Diagnosis of haemochromatosis should only be made after exclusion of other entities associated with T2 shortening of the pituitary gland (see differential diagnosis). In this case, the skull base also showed hypointense signal in both T2 and T2*, probably caused by medullary iron deposition, and with maintained contours of the gland and sella, space-occupying lesions are highly unlikely (◨ Fig. 66.4). Given the patient's history, it is reasonable to assert that the hypopituitarism is caused by secondary haemochromatosis. Chelation therapy is required to prevent long-term sequelae [1]. Hormonal replacement therapy is required because of the hypopituitarism [1].

References

1. Ling CC. Panhypopituitarism in a patient with thalassemia intermedia. J ASEAN Fed Endocr Soc. 2014;26(1):65–6.
2. Sondag MJ, Wattamwar AS, Aleppo G, Nemeth AJ. Hereditary hemochromatosis. Radiology. 2012;262:1037–41.

Case 67

Daniel Dias

© Springer International Publishing AG 2018
J. Xavier et al. (eds.), *Diagnostic and Therapeutic Neuroradiology*,
https://doi.org/10.1007/978-3-319-61140-2_67

67

A 56-year-old patient with a history of anterior communicating artery aneurysm, HCV+. Asymptomatic. Admitted for a follow-up CT angiogram.

? Questions

1. What are the findings?
2. Which vascular territories are involved?
3. Which differentials could be considered?

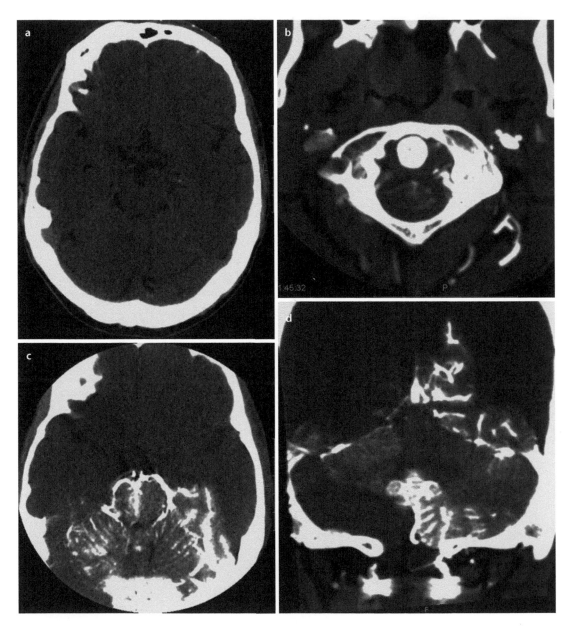

◘ Fig. 67.1   a Non enhanced CT scan; **b, c** and **d** post contrast CT scans

Diagnosis   Pseudopathologic brain parenchymal enhancement

✅ **Answers**

1. Abnormal cortical enhancement of occipital, parietal, and cerebellar cortices; sulcal/pial enhancement; and prominent vascular structures in posterior fossa (◻ Fig. 67.1c, d).
2. The vertebrobasilar territory is involved, most strikingly the left PCA (◻ Fig. 67.1d), right SCA (◻ Fig. 67.1c), and left PICA (◻ Fig. 67.1d), and filling of cervical veins and dural sinuses (◻ Fig. 67.1b, d).
3. Meningioangiomatosis, vertebrobasilar ischemia, and AVM could be considered.

67.1   Comments

Retrograde flow of contrast into the jugular veins, vertebral veins, vertebral venous plexus, and dural venous sinuses is well documented in the literature and is particularly related to left-sided venous injection for cross-sectional angiographic studies.

Cervical venous reflux can be potentiated by conditions leading to compression of the left brachiocephalic vein, phase of respiration during contrast injection, incompetent venous valves (long-standing severe tricuspid regurgitation, thoracoabdominal trauma), increased intrathoracic pressure, occlusion or stenosis of the superior vena cava, and congestive cardiac failure.

In this case, a very early acquisition after venous bolus injection showed retrograde flow into the left jugular vein and intracranial venous system (◻ Fig. 67.1c, d), with reflux through the transverse and sigmoid sinuses into the intracranial and cervical venous system (◻ Fig. 67.1b), overwhelming vascular autoregulation and leading to parenchymal enhancement.

A repeated acquisition showed rapid disappearance of the abnormal findings, excluding other potential differential diagnosis (◻ Fig. 67.2a, b).

Failure to recognize this artifact can lead to incorrect diagnosis and additional unnecessary imaging work-up. For this reason, right-sided venous injection of contrast should be preferred.

67

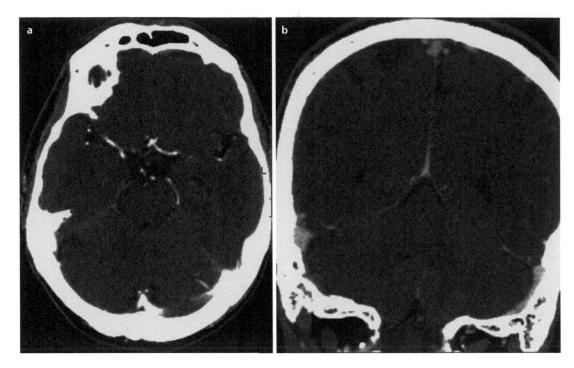

◘ Fig. 67.2   **a** Post-contrast CT scan, **b** post-contrast CT scan

References

1. Chen JY, Mamourian AC, Messe SR, Wolf RL. Pseudopathologic brain parenchymal enhancement due to venous reflux from left-sided injection and
   brachiocephalic vein narrowing. AJNR Am J Neuroradiol. 2010;31(1):86–7.
2. Tseng YC, Hsu HL, Lee TH, Chen CJ. Venous reflux on carotid computed
   tomography angiography: relationship with left-arm injection. J Comput
   Assist Tomogr. 2007;31(3):360–4.
3. Takhtani D. CT neuroangiography: a glance at the common pitfalls and
   their prevention. AJR Am J Roentgenol. 2005;185(3):772–83.

Case 68

Teresa Caixeiro

© Springer International Publishing AG 2018
J. Xavier et al. (eds.), *Diagnostic and Therapeutic Neuroradiology*,
https://doi.org/10.1007/978-3-319-61140-2_68

A 40-year-old man with recurrent headaches.

? **Questions**
1. What are the findings?
2. What is the diagnosis?

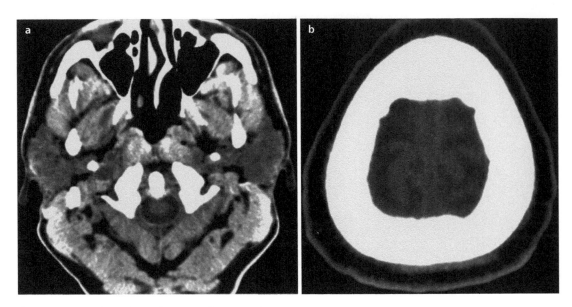

◘ Fig. 68.1   Axial unenhanced computed tomography

Diagnosis   Severe anemia

✅ **Answers to Questions**

1. The computed tomography (■ Fig. 68.1) showed hypodensity of the cerebral venous sinuses and the carotid arteries.
2. Severe anemia.

68.1   Comments

The attenuation of blood on CT is primarily a function of the protein fraction of hemoglobin [1, 2]. There is a relationship between CT attenuation and hemoglobin levels (in this case, it is 5.4 g/dl) [2].

Very low hemoglobin levels cause decreased attenuation of blood less dense than the brain on CT imaging and being responsible for the hypodensity demonstrated by vascular structures (■ Fig. 68.1) [1].

In cases with elevated hematocrit (e.g., polycythemia), CT imaging may demonstrate hyperdensity within the cerebral vasculature [2].

References

1. Lee SY, Cha SH, Lee SH, Dong-Ick Shin. Evaluation of the effect of hemoglobin or hematocrit level on dural sinus density using unenhanced computed tomography. Departments of Radiology and Neurology/College of Medicine/Chungbuk National University, Cheongju; 2013.
2. Beal JC, Overby P, Korey SR. Severe anemia leading to hypodensity of cerebral venous sinuses on computed tomography imaging. Department of Neurology/Albert Einstein College of Medicine/ Montefiore Medical Center, Bronx, NY; 2012.

Case 69

Maria Goreti Sá and José Eduardo Alves

© Springer International Publishing AG 2018
J. Xavier et al. (eds.), *Diagnostic and Therapeutic Neuroradiology*,
https://doi.org/10.1007/978-3-319-61140-2_69

A 46-year-old male, submitted, in 2005, to right hemilaminectomies at L2–L3 and L3–L4 levels due to disk herniations, with a good clinical outcome. Five years after the procedure, the patient began to complain of local, severe, lower back pain. There were no associated motor or sensory deficits.

Physical examination showed localized tenderness at the incision site, without swelling or erythema. There were no signs of radiculopathy.

? Questions

1. What are the imaging findings?
2. What are the possible differential diagnoses?
3. Which would be the next most valuable study?

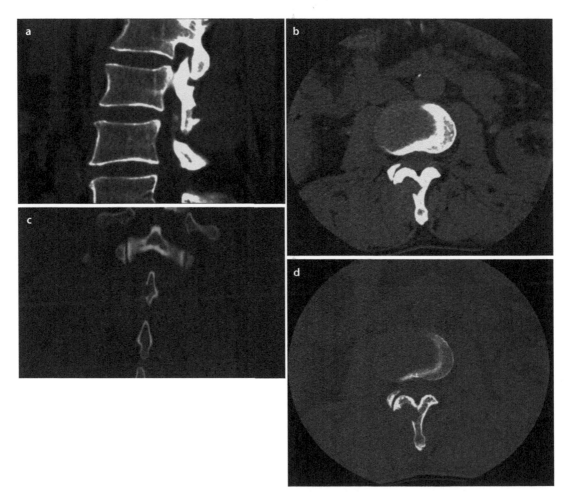

◻ Fig. 69.1   a–d CT scan images

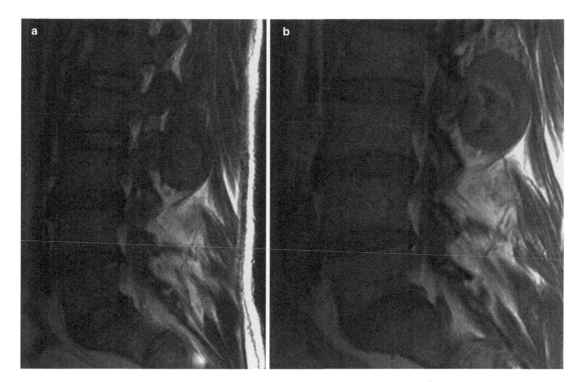

Fig. 69.2 **a, b** Sagittal T1-weighted images, before **a** and after **b** gadolinium

Diagnosis Textiloma, foreign body granuloma

✓ **Answers**

1. CT scans show a right paraspinal soft tissue mass at the L2–L3 level, isodense to the surrounding muscles (■ Fig. 69.1a); bone CT scans demonstrate invasion/destruction of the L3 spinal process by the mass (■ Fig. 69.1b–d), suggesting an aggressive lesion.

   T2-weighted MR images reveal a well-defined oval mass with heterogeneous signal: it presents a central hypointense "core", an intermediate irregular hyperintense rim, and a more peripheral low-signal intensity component (■ Fig. 69.2a).

   Contrast-enhanced T1-weighted MR images show the lesion has peripheral heterogeneous enhancement around a central non-enhancing area (■ Fig. 69.2b).

2. Foreign body granuloma, textiloma, and spinal tumor, namely, sarcoma abscess.

3. Biopsy revealed chronic inflammatory infiltration with granuloma formation and the presence of a cotton material.

69

69.1 Comments

The retention of foreign materials in surgical wounds can present either acutely, with abscess formation and delayed healing, or chronically, eliciting a granulomatous inflammatory reaction that may remain clinically silent for many years [1].

In our case, it presented as a mass lesion with bone destruction 5 years after surgery, mimicking a spinal tumor.

Although an underreported surgical complication, textiloma should be considered in the differential diagnosis when a mass is detected within a previous surgical field [1–2].

References

1. Hakan T, et al. Clinical, pathological and radiological features of paraspinal textiloma: report of two cases and review of the literature. Neurol Neurochir Pol. 2009;43(5):475–8.
2. Okten, et al. Textiloma: a case of foreign body mimicking a spinal mass. Eur Spine J. 2006;15(Suppl. 5):S626–9.

Case 70

Teresa Caixeiro

© Springer International Publishing AG 2018
J. Xavier et al. (eds.), *Diagnostic and Therapeutic Neuroradiology*,
https://doi.org/10.1007/978-3-319-61140-2_70

A 20-month-old child is referred with right-sided leucocoria.

❓ Questions
1. What is the most likely diagnosis?
2. Which entities should be included in differential diagnosis?

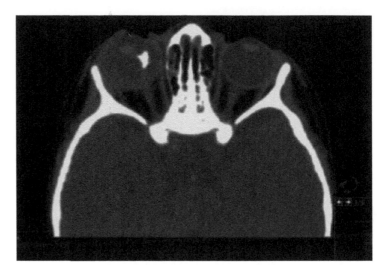

◘ Fig. 70.1   Axial unenhanced CT

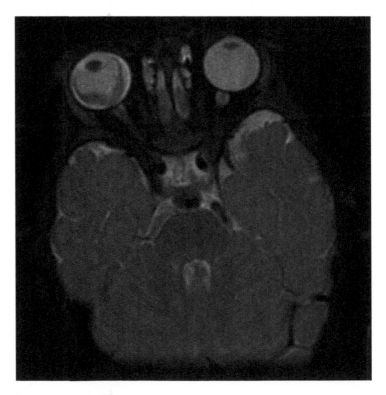

◘ Fig. 70.2   Axial T2

Case 70

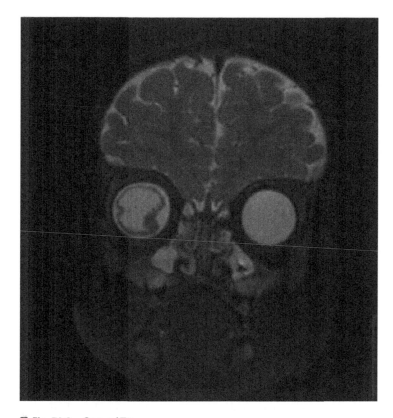

■ **Fig. 70.3** Coronal T2

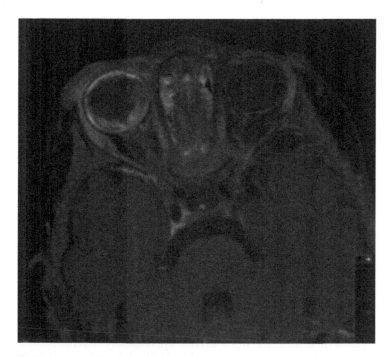

■ **Fig. 70.4** Postcontrast axial T1 fat sat

Diagnosis   Retinoblastoma

✓ **Answers to questions**
1. Retinoblastoma.
2. Several conditions may mimic retinoblastomas such as Coats' disease, retinopathy of prematurity, premature retinopathy, persistent hyperplastic vitreous humour, and Toxocara canis endophthalmitis. None of these conditions, however, have calcification in the early stages.

70.1 Comments

Retinoblastoma is the most common intraocular childhood tumour with 95% of cases developing before the age of 5 [1]. Retinoblastoma may be sporadic or secondary to a germline mutation of the RB tumour suppressor gene which is usually inherited. It may be unilateral or bilateral:

- Bilateral tumours (30–40% of cases) essentially always have a germline mutation.
- Unilateral tumours (60–70% of cases) are caused by a germline mutation in approximately 15% of cases, whereas 85% of cases are sporadic. Thus, 55% of cases are due to a germline mutation.

Retinoblastomas may involve the vitreous humour, lymphatics, or along the optic nerve into the brain or into the subarachnoid space resulting in leptomeningeal metastases. In rare germline cases, there may be a trilateral tumour (bilateral retinoblastoma and pineoblastoma) and osteosarcoma. These cases have a poor prognosis, making an early diagnosis very important.

Common presentations of retinoblastomas include leucocoria, strabismus, decreased vision (particularly in bilateral lesions), retinal detachment, glaucoma, ocular pain, or signs of ocular inflammation.

The CT typically shows enhanced calcified retinal masses. The calcification is commonly punctate or clumped (◻ Fig. 70.1). MR imaging is also found to be useful in the follow-up of these patients. The tumour is typically hyperintense relative to the vitreous humour on T1-weighted and proton density images and is hypointense on T2-weighted images [1] (◻ Figs. 70.2 and 70.3).

CT is better at detecting calcification than MR, whereas contrast-enhanced MR (◻ Fig. 70.4) is more sensitive than CT for detecting tumoural extension into the nerve and intracranial space and for detecting secondary lesions [2].

Treatment options depend on the bulk of the disease (MRI being the modality of choice for the pretreatment staging of retinoblastoma). These include enucleation (surgical removal of the eye), radiotherapy, chemotherapy, photocoagulation, and cryotherapy. In bilateral disease, the worst affected eye is usually enucleated, and the contralateral eye receives other treatment options, such as radiotherapy, in order to salvage sight.

References

1. Rauschecker AM, Patel CV, Yeom KW, Eisenhut CA, Gawande RS, O'Brien JM, Ebrahimi KB, Daldrup-Link HE. High-resolution MR imaging of the orbit in patients with retinoblastoma. Radiographics. 2012;32(5):1307–26. https://doi.org/10.1148/rg.325115176.
2. Yousem DM, Grossman RI. Neuroradiology, the requisites. 3rd ed, 2010.

Supplementary Information

Index – 383

Index

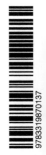